Introduction to
Biosocial Medicine

Introduction to Biosocial Medicine

The Social, Psychological, and Biological Determinants of Human Behavior and Well-Being

Donald A. Barr, MD, PhD

JOHNS HOPKINS UNIVERSITY PRESS
Baltimore

Johns Hopkins University Press
2715 North Charles Street
Baltimore, Maryland 21218-4363
www.press.jhu.edu

Library of Congress Cataloging-in-Publication Data

Barr, Donald A., author.
   Introduction to biosocial medicine : the social, psychological, and biological
determinants of human behavior and well-being / Donald A. Barr.
         p. ; cm.
   Includes bibliographical references and index.
   ISBN 978-1-4214-1860-5 (pbk. : alk. paper)—ISBN 1-4214-1860-6 (pbk. : alk.
paper)—ISBN 978-1-4214-1861-2 (electronic)—ISBN 1-4214-1861-4 (electronic)
   I. Title.
   [DNLM: 1. Behavioral Medicine—education. 2. Social Medicine—education.
3. Socioeconomic Factors. WA 31]
   RA418
   362.1—dc23   2015008457

A catalog record for this book is available from the British Library.

Figures 8.3, 8.5, 8.6, 8.7, 8.8, 8.11, 8.12 by Jacqueline Schaffer

*Special discounts are available for bulk purchases of this book. For more information,
please contact Special Sales at 410-516-6936 or specialsales@press.jhu.edu.*

Johns Hopkins University Press uses environmentally friendly book materials,
including recycled text paper that is composed of at least 30 percent post-
consumer waste, whenever possible.

For Deagon

Thus, the determinants of health are best conceptualized as biosocial *phenomena, in which health and disease emerge through the interaction between biology and the social environment.*

—Michael Westerhaus, Amy Finnegan, Mona Haidar, Arthur Kleinman, Joia Mukherjee, and Paul Farmer, "The Necessity of Social Medicine in Medical Education," *Academic Medicine,* 2015

Contents

Preface

For more than twenty years, I have been affiliated with the Program in Human Biology at Stanford University. I teach undergraduate courses on health policy and health disparities and advise numerous undergraduates who are heading in different professional directions, nearly all of whom want to focus their careers on improving human well-being.

The Program in Human Biology at Stanford was founded in 1971 by a team of scientists from a range of academic backgrounds, including biology, genetics, psychology, sociology, pediatrics, and psychiatry. The intent behind the creation of Human Biology as Stanford's first interdisciplinary program of studies available to undergraduates is described in comments by Gordon Harrison of the Ford Foundation, which provided an initial grant to establish the Stanford program: "It is a rare sociologist today who has had even one course in biology; it is still rarer for an economist or political scientist. Study of the behavior of people has traditionally been fragmented. Many biologists, meanwhile, have acted as though evolution stopped at the lower primates" (Program in Human Biology, p. 2). From its inception, the Program in Human Biology has combined the study of the biology of humans with that of the social and psychological aspects of human behavior. In doing so it has attempted to break down the intellectual boundaries that so often separate academic disciplines. It has since grown to be one of the largest undergraduate majors at Stanford.

The intellectual home provided by Human Biology turned out to be a good fit for me. I am that "rare sociologist who has ever had a course in biology." After earning my MD and practicing medicine for fifteen years, I returned to Stanford and earned my PhD in sociology in 1993. Since then I have focused my research, writing, and teaching at the intersection of biological, social, and behavioral sciences, emphasizing the importance of this interdisciplinary approach as a preparation for a range of professional careers having to do with human health and well-being.

We know now that the founders of Human Biology were prescient in their approach to learning. Research in the human genome has linked patterns of genetic variation to a range of human behavioral characteristics and health outcomes. In parallel, a growing body of research has shown that factors in the social and psychological environment of infants and children can change the way in which genetic information is expressed, leading to measurable differences in neural structure and physiologic functioning that can last a lifetime. It seems an appropriate time to offer a new text linking human behavior to human well-being by integrating a range of academic perspectives.

Two other developments, unrelated to each other, reinforce the appropriateness of the timing for a new approach to teaching about this topic. The first is the rapid movement at universities such as Stanford to online learning and the various web-based approaches to teaching associated with that movement. These include MOOCs (massive open online courses) as well as the flipped classroom, "in which students absorb an instructor's lecture in a digital format as homework, freeing up class time for a focus on applications, including emotion-provoking simulation exercises" (Prober and Heath 2012, p. 1658).

If a lecture I give to my class changes little from year to year, why not simply record the lecture and make it available online for students to watch as their homework? We can then use classroom time to engage in a discussion of the concepts and unanswered questions raised in the online lecture and associated readings. As Prober and Heath describe, with the flipped classroom, "teachers would be able to actually teach, rather than merely make speeches." I hope to create a series of recorded lectures in which I cover much of the material in this book, but from more of an analytic and questioning perspective. If we are studying learned behavior using a chapter from this text, in a web lecture I might discuss the question of the extent to which "learning" actually involves changes to brain structure, as compared to creating new patterns of memory that don't alter brain structure. This will give us the opportunity to discuss in class which perspective seems to be the most consistent with available evidence and what types of new research questions might need to be addressed to resolve any differences in perspective. As others also develop web-based learning resources that cover aspects of human behavior and human well-being, I hope this text might provide a useful supplement to those resources.

A second important development has been the decision by the Association of American Medical Colleges (AAMC) to change the format of the Medical College Admission Test (MCAT), required of most applicants to medical school in the United States. The epigraph to this book is from a commentary published in 2015 in the journal *Academic Medicine* by a group of national leaders in the field of social medicine (Westerhaus et al. 2015). In their commentary these authors argue that "medical education requires a comprehensive transformation to incorporate rigorous biosocial training to ensure that all future health professionals are equipped with the knowledge and skills necessary to practice social medicine." With a growing recognition that physicians need to understand the biosocial sciences behind human behavior in order to be effective practitioners, in 2015 the MCAT added a new test section titled "The Psychological, Social, and Biological Foundations of Behavior," testing students' competency in core aspects of biosocial medicine.

The AAMC reported that in 2012, more than 45,000 individuals applied to medical school in the United States. That number is expected to grow in the future. Nearly all of these applicants will be asked to develop an understanding of human behavior as part of their undergraduate preparation. Undergraduate colleges and universities, however, do not have consistent curricular offerings in this area. Although it is not my intent to offer this book as a simple "MCAT Prep" tool, I nonetheless want to provide an educational resource that will be useful for students looking to acquire an understanding of the complex roots of human behavior. I hope this book can contribute to this goal while maintaining a level of scholarship appropriate for use in teaching at colleges and universities.

REFERENCES

Association of American Medical Colleges. US medical school applicants and students 1982-1983 to 2011-2012, available at www.aamc.org/download /153708/data/charts1982to2012.pdf, accessed 6/8/13.

Prober, C. G., & Heath, C. 2012. Lecture halls without lectures: A proposal for medical education. New England Journal of Medicine 366: 1657-59.

Program in Human Biology, Stanford University. The first 30 years, available at https://humbio.stanford.edu/sites/default/files/alumni_/humbiohistory.pdf, accessed 6/8/13.

Westerhaus, M., Finnegan, A., Haidar, M., Kleinman, A., Mukherjee, M., & Farmer, P. 2015. The necessity of social medicine in medical education. Academic Medicine. doi: 10.1097/ACM.

Introduction to Biosocial Medicine

Understanding Human Behavior

It seems self-evident to suggest that human well-being is closely tied to human behavior. In order to improve well-being, logic would suggest, we need simply to change unhealthy behavior. Those who have worked in health care, in education, or in similar fields for which improving well-being is the principal professional goal will tell you that this is no simple task.

It is often intensely frustrating to work with an individual who is engaging in a behavior that directly harms that individual's own well-being. Cigarette smoking provides an example. For decades, doctors and smokers alike have known of the direct causal link between smoking, heart disease, lung cancer, and emphysema—and yet, inciting a smoker to quit can be one of the most difficult challenges a physician or other health professional can confront.

"Behavior patterns represent the single most prominent domain of influence over health prospects in the United States." These were the words McGinnis and colleagues used in 2002 (p. 82) to underscore just how necessary human behaviors are to well-being. Building on McGinnis's data, Schroeder (2007) estimated that of the many deaths that occur prematurely in the United States, 40 percent are directly attributable to behavioral patterns, chief among them smoking, obesity and inactivity, and alcohol use. As Schroeder describes, "The single greatest opportunity to improve health and reduce premature deaths lies in personal behavior" (p. 1222).

The need to understand human behavior

If human well-being is linked inextricably to behavior, it becomes essential for those who will spend their professional career working to improve well-being to gain a fundamental understanding of just what behavior is in the human context and what factors influence behavior. This book is written to enhance this understanding. I intend the book to be used as part of a course at the college or university level to provide students—both those with a clear professional trajectory ahead of them and those who haven't yet decided the direction their career will take—with an understanding of the many different factors that can act singly or in concert to affect how people behave.

Those who have spent time at a college or university are well aware that different academic disciplines often adopt differing perspectives on topics of common interest, such as human behavior. Psychology—defined by the American Psychological Association as "the study of the mind and behavior"—explores the development of the human mind from its biological roots through birth, childhood, and adulthood. The work of psychologists overlaps with that of sociologists, who define their field as engaged in "the scientific study of society, including patterns of social relationships, social interaction, and culture" (American Sociological Association). Clearly these broad social forces can have powerful influences on how individuals behave.

From a different perspective, though, one can argue that behavior only happens when nerves within the human brain respond to sensory input to initiate neural messages to the muscles and other organs that control human action. It is hard to argue with the assertion that, at its very core, behavior is biological in nature.

I hope the reader will see that each of these perspectives—the biological, the psychological, and the sociological—has value, but that none can alone give us the full understanding of the determinants of human behavior that we need in order to address behavior and its consequences in a professional capacity. To understand behavior, we need to cross over traditional disciplinary boundaries, and view behavior as multifactorial, with roots in the biology of neurons, the human mind, and the influence of broad social forces on individual perceptions and responses. This is the approach I take in this book.

What is behavior?

One way to answer this question is to look to a dictionary for a definition of *behavior*. The Oxford English Dictionary provides such a definition as the "manner of conducting oneself in the external relations of life . . . The manner in which a thing acts under specified conditions or circumstances, or in relation to other things." A somewhat more vernacular definition is provided by Wikipedia, which describes behavior as "the response of the system or organism to various stimuli or inputs, whether internal or external, conscious or subconscious, overt or covert, and voluntary or involuntary." Behavior, it seems, is how we act in response to external factors.

Another way to understand the meaning of behavior is to move beyond formal definitions and instead to describe a range of different behaviors common to humans. We can then consider what these various patterns of human responses and actions may have in common, and in so doing arrive at a more functional definition of 'behavior.'

The first behavior I will consider is that described above: smoking cigarettes. As we know (or should know), "smoking causes lung cancer, heart disease, emphysema, and may complicate pregnancy"—as stated in the warning prominently displayed on packages of cigarettes sold in the United States, as required by federal law (US Code, Section 1333). This warning is intended to target the individual about to light up a cigarette, with the hopes of discouraging the smoker by describing the proven health risk. This approach seems to assume that the decision to smoke a cigarette is made consciously by an individual after balancing risks and benefits. However, data in figure 1.1 convey a different message.

The chart shows the percentage of US adults who were current smokers in 2011, sorted by gender and educational attainment, as reported by the federal government (US Centers for Disease Control and Prevention 2012). There is a clear and continuous educational gradient in the

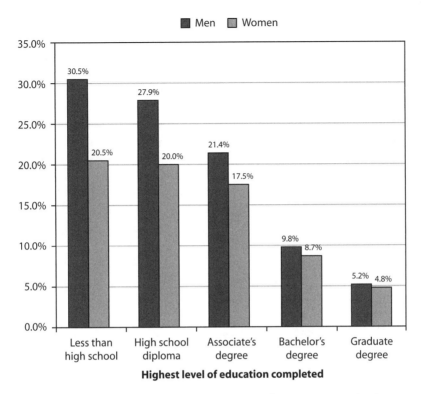

■ Men ■ Women

FIGURE 1.1. Percentage of Persons Age ≥18 Years Who Were Current Smokers, 2011. US Centers for Disease Control and Prevention, MMWR 2012: 61(44):889-94.

association between smoking prevalence and education, and a consistent gender difference. The more education one completes, the less likely one is to smoke. At all levels of education, women are less likely to smoke than men.

Most of the education reported in figure 1.1 is completed by the age of 25, yet the association between smoking and education persists throughout the adult years. This association of both education and gender with a behavior with clear harm to well-being suggests that not all behavior is simply the result of individual choice. Given that "smoking and high blood pressure . . . are responsible for the largest number of deaths in the US" (Danaei et al. 2009, p. 1), it would appear that behavior at the individual level is influenced by broader social forces and has profound impacts on the overall well-being of our society.

If education is so closely linked to behaviors such as smoking that affect well-being, what might be the factors that affect education? As with smoking, on the surface one's behavior regarding education would seem to be based on choices made by the individual: Shall I work hard in this class? Shall I do my homework? Shall I study for the exam? Educational attainment, often measured as the number of years of schooling completed or the highest degree obtained, has a powerful association with well-being throughout life. Yet educational attainment does not follow a pattern suggestive of individual choice as the driving force.

An excellent example of this is provided in work done by Dubow and colleagues (2009). They used data from a study that followed children in a semirural area of New York state from when the children were 8 years old until they were 48. They looked at a range of factors during the subjects' younger years that predicted the level of education they had attained by age 48, including things such as socioeconomic status, childhood IQ, and childhood behavior. They found that the educational attainment of the children's parents when the children were 8 years old was one of the strongest predictors of eventual educational attainment when the children had grown to be 48 years old.

An especially interesting aspect of this association is that it seemed to be indirect—that is, it happened in a two-step process. The principal impact of the parents' level of educational attainment at the time the child was 8 years old was to affect the child's educational aspirations as an adolescent: the higher the parents' education, the greater the adolescent's aspirations to succeed in his or her education. It was those adolescent aspirations that seemed to drive the child's eventual educational attainment as an adult. The home educational environment in which a child grows up seems to have powerful effects on that child's aspiration for and success in educational attainment.

The work of Mischel and colleagues (1988) suggests that a child's perspective on attaining educational success may be powerfully affected by psychological characteristics already in place at age 4. Mischel offered a group of 4-year-old preschool children the alternatives of playing patiently with toys for about fifteen minutes to attain a two-marshmallow reward, versus asking for a one-marshmallow reward without having to wait. Mischel then followed these children into adolescence and found that those children who as 4-year-olds chose to wait were, as adolescents, "more academically and socially competent, verbally fluent, rational, attentive, planful, and able to deal well with frustration and stress" (p. 687).

If 4-year-olds show differential patterns of response to external factors, will younger children also do so? How about newborn infants? Might they exhibit differential patterns of response to

stimuli? Moon and colleagues (2013) played recordings of vowel sounds to newborns less than two days old. Some of the sounds were taken from the mother's native language and some from a nonnative language. The infants wore pacifiers that sensed how often they sucked. The researchers found that infants sucked more slowly in response to native sounds than to nonnative ones, leading the authors to conclude that "birth is not a benchmark that reflects a complete separation between the effects of nature versus those of nurture . . . neonates' perception of speech sounds already reflects some degree of learning" (p. 159).

Looking across these various studies, and using smoking as one example of human behavior, we see that

- one's propensity to smoke as an adult is powerfully associated with one's level of education;
- one's level of education is associated with the strength of one's educational aspirations as an adolescent;
- one's educational aspirations as an adolescent are associated with the level of education attained by one's parents when one is an 8-year-old;
- one's educational attainment as an adolescent is also associated with one's ability as a 4-year-old to delay gratification; and
- newborn infants display differential patterns of sucking on a pacifier in response to sounds reminiscent of the mother's voice, presumably heard while *in utero*.

Each of these behaviors is a pattern of response to external stimuli. The stimulus may be a cigarette waiting to be lit, a homework assignment waiting to be completed, a parental attitude regarding the value of education, a choice between differential rewards, or simply a sound one hears. Each behavior involves a stimulus and a response, presumably mediated by our interpretation of the stimulus.

Based on these repeating patterns, I suggest that behavior has three core components:

1. our perception of external stimuli;
2. our interpretation of those stimuli; and
3. our response to that interpretation.

This is how I approach the concept of human behavior throughout this book. I have laid out the chapters of the book accordingly.

Well-being and the consequences of behavior (chapter 2)

Having laid out the steps of the behavioral process—perception, interpretation, and response—I turn to the growing body of evidence that links behavior to many different types of well-being. One way of viewing well-being is from the perspective of life expectancy and the frequency of potentially preventable deaths. Researchers have estimated that nearly half of preventable deaths are a direct consequence of specific behaviors, principal among them smoking, diet, and alcohol abuse.

In addition to the length of life, well-being also has a great deal to do with the quality of life. We will consider the growing evidence that variations in one's perceptions of well-being often have psychological and linked behavioral roots. As with many physical behaviors, these perceptions are often strongly associated with one's level of educational attainment.

Well-being also has to do with the strength of the personal and social connections we make with others. Our cognition and our sense of self will affect how we respond to others around us and in so doing will help determine the level of support we experience from others. The strength of our social networks and social support have repeatedly been shown to affect both physical and psychological well-being. This is true both for those in our family and those we interact with who are not. At its essence, well-being has to do with the quality of our life as we perceive

it. Much of that quality of life is directly affected by our own patterns of behavior.

The impact of social inequality and social hierarchy on behavior (chapter 3)

One of the most powerful stressors a person can face, either as a child or as an adult, is social inequality. Social inequality has been shown to be associated with a range of behaviors that are central to well-being. This chapter considers the forms social inequality can take and the ways these forms can overlap.

Central to our understanding of broader social inequality is economic inequality. Being born into a low-income family exposes a child to very real physical and environmental factors that can be harmful to child development and well-being. From air quality and housing quality to the quality of the local food environment, those in a position of economic disadvantage will often experience a disadvantaged physical environment as well.

The social environment of economic inequality can also have powerful effects. One's position on the economic hierarchy often conveys symbolic messages about one's position in the hierarchy of social structure, with those lower on the structural hierarchy having fewer opportunities to raise their position.

Concurrent with economic inequality, most societies also experience inequality based on race or ethnicity. The racial or ethnic group with which one identifies can have an important influence on one's perception of self. Our race or ethnicity can also create powerful perceptions among others about who we are, how we are expected to behave, and how we are to be treated by others. This level of inequality can be based either on race or on ethnicity—two categories that overlap yet have significant distinguishing characteristics. I will describe race both as a biological concept and as a social construct.

There are fundamental shifts taking place in the demographics of the US population. Many among the growing number of Hispanics in this country do not identify with a racial group separate from their Hispanic heritage. As per US Census Bureau policies, Hispanic is considered an ethnicity, while white, black, Asian, Native American, and Native Hawaiian are considered to be races. Accordingly, in using *Hispanic*, I will mean someone of any race who is also Hispanic. In addition, I refer to the US Census category of "Black or African American" by the shortened term of *black*. When I use terms such as *white* and *black*, I refer to those who are of the white or black race and are not Hispanic. It is certainly possible for those who are Hispanic also to have a racial identity. However, in looking at the dynamics of the US population in terms of behavior and well-being, I find it most useful and informative to refer to Hispanics of any race as a single category.

However race and ethnicity are defined, they often lead to levels of social inequality that subsume economic inequality as well as other forms of social disadvantage. The use of racial stereotypes is a principal contributor to this inequality. These stereotypes are often invoked unconsciously, either by a person of a majority racial group interacting with a member of a racial minority or by a member of a minority group himself or herself when assessing self-efficacy or other similar characteristics. The combination of racial inequality and economic inequality can have profound adverse impacts both on behavior and on well-being, impacts that can persist across generations.

Any discussion of inequality should also consider gender inequality and the impacts it can have on self-perception and behavior. Clearly, some aspects of gendered behavior are a result of biological differences between males and females. Gendered aspects of one's personality as well as learned behavior may, by contrast, have little to do with biology and a great deal to do with how we are treated by others.

How cultural context affects behavior (chapter 4)

As we develop psychologically from birth, we become aware of, interact with, and respond to a growing network of other people. Assuming that our mother is our primary caregiver after birth, she is often the first "other" we recognize. Gradually we come to recognize other family members and begin to adapt both our sense of identity and our patterns of behavior to those around us. (For me as a young child, it didn't take long to learn from my older brother that he was the *big* brother and I was the *little* brother, and I was expected to behave accordingly.)

As we grow and mature, our social environment grows to include peers and others who make up our community, however we come to understand that concept. That sense of community may carry with it a clear sense of status ordering and of which groups are dominant. As part of our growing identification with a community, we may also begin to develop a sense of ethnicity and culture, both of which can carry expectations of beliefs and behaviors. As we mature we become aware that our family and our community exist within the context of a broader society. We also become aware of the various and sometimes conflicting norms and behavioral expectations the broader social order may apply.

From this increasingly complex set of social influences, we adapt both our ways of thinking and our sense of self. As we use our cognitive abilities and our personality to interpret the things we see, hear, and otherwise perceive, we adapt our behaviors so as to fit in to the social and cultural context in which we live—that is, unless we become a nonconformist, rejecting the dominant social and cultural norms and behaving based on our own, internalized values. Such a response can often be perceived negatively by those around us; sometimes, however, it is instead perceived as innovative or creative and is received positively by others.

Social group identity, status inequality, and behavior (chapter 5)

As children move into adolescence and adulthood, they become increasingly aware of the attitudes and behaviors of those immediately around them. While adolescents and young adults continue to perceive themselves to be part of a broad social or cultural group, they come increasingly to identify with a specific group or groups as well as identifying those groups of which they are not members. They will often compare themselves to those around them based on their perceived level of capital, measured in economic, cultural, and social terms.

Sometimes people find themselves around others they don't know. How a person responds to an interaction with another person may depend on how he or she explains to himself or herself that individual's motivations—even if that attribution proves not to be accurate. How one perceives others can also affect how that individual responds to certain unexpected circumstances, such as another person's need for assistance. In a similar manner, in many Western cultures, working on a task as a member of a group, rather than as an individual, will often affect the level of effort one exerts, as compared to the situation in which one works alone on the task. Becoming aware of the ways in which social context can influence behavior is especially important to our overall understanding of human behavior.

Motivation as a key mediator of behavior (chapter 6)

Once we have perceived the stimuli confronting us in our physical and social environment and interpreted those stimuli in the context of the ways we have learned to think and the person whom we perceive ourselves to be, the next step is to decide how to act in response. Our motivation is the link between perception and action. Motivation involves a complex array of biological and psychological factors. Feeling hungry—a process triggered by certain biochemical messengers linking the digestive system and the brain—gives us the message that we should find something to eat. Feeling cold—another biological process triggered by messages between sensors in the periphery of the body and the thermostat situated in the hypothalamus of our brain—gives us the message to do something to get warmer. Perhaps we should put on a sweater, or perhaps we should turn up the heat in our home. Feeling cold is the motivation for taking some action to get warmer.

Sexual arousal in response to viewing someone we perceive as attractive certainly has a powerful biological component, but that response is mixed with concepts of appropriate and inappropriate behavior we have internalized from our social and cultural surroundings. Similarly, feeling angry and wanting to respond accordingly reflects a motivation derived from our interpretation of what we have seen, heard, or felt.

One of the principal theories of how various factors affect our motivation and our responses is provided by the concept of the "hierarchy of needs" proposed by psychologist Abraham Maslow (1943). According to this hierarchy, we respond first to core physiologic needs, such as hunger and the need for sleep. As we are able to address basic needs, we move on to those on the next step of the hierarchy: feeling safe and feeling as though we belong in our family or social group. Eventually we move to what Maslow referred to as "self-actualization"—working to fulfill our hopes and aspirations for a meaningful life.

As one might imagine, establishing and responding to our own hierarchy involves negotiating the ways family, peers, community, and society affect how we interpret our situation and how we choose to respond. Often motivation becomes a question of meeting our own expectations for ourselves versus meeting the expectation others have placed upon us. A student might know that his or her parents want him or her to be good at math and to go to a good college but that he or she really loves music, especially the way he or she feels when playing jazz. How does this student balance all of this in developing his or her own motives for action? An important part of these types of decisions has to do with time perspective. Are we motivated to act for an immediate outcome, or are we instead acting so as to attain a more distant outcome some time in the future? As we will see, the motivation to succeed in school can be powerfully affected by our time perspective.

Personality: Who we are (chapter 7)

As we grow as children and begin to recognize and respond to an increasingly complex array or patterns and relationships, we also begin to develop a sense of who we are as distinct from those around us. We begin to develop a "personality." Scientists have been studying the nature of human personality for more than a century. At the turn of the 20th century, Sigmund Freud proposed his theory of psychosexual development, suggesting that we develop the core aspects of our personality in early childhood and describing five specific stages of that development. By contrast, Erik Erikson described eight stages of personality development and suggested that the process continues throughout our lives.

It seems clear that, whatever the timing and staging, each of us develops certain key personality characteristics. Some psychologists refer to "the Big Five," describing people in terms of five central characteristics: openness, conscientiousness, extroversion, agreeableness, and neuroticism. Different aspects of these characteristics in different combinations can provide a sense of identity and can help us to prioritize our goals and select our actions. How we express and act on these characteristics will also

provide others around us with a sense of who we are and how we are likely to respond to different circumstances.

We have come to recognize certain psychological characteristics as abnormal. I conclude this chapter with a description of some of the most important types of psychological disorders as well as a discussion of the extent to which these disorders may have a biological basis.

Neural structure as a basis of behavior (chapter 8)

In this chapter I describe, in terms easily understood by nonneuroanatomists, the structure of the brain, the peripheral nervous system, and the autonomic nervous system. Using the basic senses (vision, hearing, etc.) as examples, I discuss how stimuli from the external environment are conveyed to the brain. I then describe some of the basic structures of the human brain and how they are connected in ways that give us, as humans, our incredible capacities for things such as language, reading, music, and love.

Next I address the issue of brain plasticity. Whereas many mammals are born with most of their neural connections intact, human infants need time to complete many of these connections. A baby giraffe can get up and walk within hours of birth—and a good thing it can, given the proximity of predators. A human infant, however, hasn't completed this brain circuitry yet—and a good thing it hasn't, because if it waited *in utero* for all these connections to mature, its head would be so large it would never make it through the mother's birth canal.

We have growing evidence that a child's brain is continuously making and remaking the nerve connections between its various parts. For example, learning to read requires developing connections between the parts of the brain that perceive vision and sound and the part of the brain that recognizes words and gives them meaning. Children in different family or social situations learn to read at different rates, implying that their brains' nerve connections are developing at different rates, often in response to external factors.

This brings us to the concept of epigenetics—the potential for the environment external to the human body to change the way human genetic information is translated into human functions and capacities. This process is especially important in our understanding of the impacts of stressful environments on developing infants, impacts that can last a lifetime and lead to reduced well-being as an adult.

Cognition: How we think and what we know (chapter 9)

Once we have gathered various sensory data into our brains, we need to connect the inputs and link them up to previous experiences in order to give them meaning. That is, we need to interpret what we have sensed—we need to think about it. Much of the process of thinking involves finding images or other types of patterns we have previously experienced and which we remember. We give the new sensory input meaning by comparing it to what we have previously encountered.

For this thinking process to occur, we must learn to make sense of what we perceive. Of course, this process starts in childhood and continues throughout much of our life. Often referred to as a child's "cognitive development", the process actually begins in utero, as suggested by the study of the sucking patterns of newborns described above. Not surprisingly, the family in which one grows up as well as the social and cultural context in which the family lives will shape the meaning we give to the thoughts we have when responding to input from our environment. Also not surprisingly, the meaning we give to these thoughts will have substantial impact on the actions we take—or don't take—in response to what we have perceived.

How social inequality and stressful childhood experiences impact cognition, behavior, and well-being (chapter 10)

Recent science has demonstrated the extent to which our perception of and response to stress is a biological process that is central to our physical existence. In the same way that the hypothalamus of our brain acts as a thermostat, directing the regulation of our body temperature, it also functions as our *allostat*, directing the regulation of our physiologic response to stress.

A growing literature looking at infancy and early childhood has provided strong evidence that the neural and biochemical components of our response to stress are influenced by the quality of the physical and social environment in which we are raised. Researchers have pointed to a "critical period" during the months following birth during which exposure to unusual stress can permanently change the neural structure of our stress response, such that throughout childhood and perhaps adulthood we experience an exaggerated production of hormonal stress responders such as epinephrine and cortisol. Chronically elevated levels of these stress hormones can affect both our cognitive processes and our cardiovascular system in ways that are potentially harmful.

Realizing that toxic levels of stress experienced in early childhood can result in both abnormal psychological responses and harmful physiological responses underscores the importance of understanding ways of intervening for children at risk so as to buffer the potentially lifelong effect of a stressful home or social environment. If education is a principal determinant of whether one smokes cigarettes as an adult and an exaggerated stress response can impede children's educational success, we may see important opportunities for early childhood intervention to avert the adverse behavioral consequences that follow from early life stressors.

Connecting the causes of early adversity to well-being over the life course: Understanding the causal links and the interventions that hold the most promise (chapter 11)

In the final chapter I emphasize how the factors discussed throughout the book, from neural structure to perceptions of inequality and stress, continuously interact to affect the way people think both about themselves and about the world they live in. Behavior is the response to these perceptions and is heavily influenced by experiences during infancy and early childhood. For those who will work in fields that address the consequences of human behavior, gaining an understanding of these many interacting factors and forces will be an important guide to our own professional behavior as well as helping us to identify those interventions that can have meaningful, long-term impact on both the behavior and the well-being of those with whom we work.

REFERENCES

American Psychological Association. How does the APA define "psychology"?, available at www.apa.org/support/about/apa/psychology.aspx#answer, accessed 4/24/13.

American Sociological Association. What is sociology?, available at www.asanet.org/introtosociology/Documents/Field%20of%20sociology033108.htm, accessed 4/24/13.

Danaei, G., Ding, E. L., Mozaffarian, D., et al. 2009. The preventable causes of death in the United States: Comparative risk assessment of dietary, lifestyle, and metabolic risk factors. PLoS Medicine 6: e1000058.

Dubow, E. F., Boxer, P., & Huesmann, L. R. 2009. Long-term effects of parents' education on children's educational and occupational success: Mediation by family interactions, child aggression, and teenage aspirations. Merrill-Palmer Quarterly 55(3): 224–49.

Maslow, A. H. 1943. A theory of human motivation. Psychological Review 50(4): 370–96.

McGinnis, J. M., Williams-Russo, P., & Knickman, J. R. 2002. The case for more active policy attention to health promotion. Health Affairs 21(2): 78–93.

Mischel, W., Shoda, Y., & Peake, P. K. 1988. The nature of adolescent competencies predicted by preschool delay of gratification. Journal of Personality and Social Psychology 54(4): 687–96.

Moon, C., Lagercrantz, H., & Kuhl, P. K. 2013. Language experienced in utero affects vowel perception after birth: A two-country study. Acta Paediatrica 102: 156–60.

Oxford English Dictionary online. Behavior, available at www.oed.com/view/Entry/17197?redirectedFrom=behavior#eid, accessed 4/24/13.

Schroeder, S. A. 2007. We can do better: Improving the health of the American people. New England Journal of Medicine 357(12): 1221–28.

US Centers for Disease Control and Prevention. 2012. Current cigarette smoking among adults—United States, 2011. Morbidity and Mortality Weekly Report 61(44): 889–94.

US Code, Section 1333: 15 U.S.C. §1333. Labeling; requirements; conspicuous statement.

Wikipedia. Behavior, available at http://en.wikipedia.org/wiki/Behavior, accessed 4/24/13.

Behavior and Well-Being

As a first step toward gaining a deeper understanding of the ways in which behavior affects well-being, we need to delineate what we mean by *well-being* and how we can evaluate the state of well-being of an individual, a social group, or a society. One of the most common ways to approach well-being is in relation to one's health status, with *health* defined largely in terms of the presence or absence of, as well as the impact of disease. Research in a range of contexts has demonstrated that, while health status and well-being are certainly closely associated, they are not synonymous. Well-being encompasses a range of factors beyond the presence or absence of disease.

In the United States, the Centers for Disease Control and Prevention (CDCP) is the principal federal agency charged with tracking and reporting the well-being of the US population. In doing this, CDCP has adopted a broad concept of well-being, stating that "There is no consensus around a single definition of well-being, but there is general agreement that at minimum, well-being includes the presence of positive emotions and moods (e.g., contentment, happiness), the absence of negative emotions (e.g., depression, anxiety), satisfaction with life, fulfillment and positive functioning." The CDCP goes on to enumerate different aspects of well-being, including:

- physical well-being,
- development and activity,
- social well-being,
- emotional well-being,
- psychological well-being, and
- economic well-being.

Researchers have identified links between behavior and many of these different approaches to well-being.

Physical well-being

In comparing the health of societies or other social groups, one of the most frequently cited measures is life expectancy. Life expectancy can be measured at various times throughout the life span and addresses the question, "on average, how many additional years will a person who has reached a certain age live?" The earliest measure is life expectancy at birth. As reported by the CDCP (2013d), in 2010, a male baby born in the United States could expect to live 76.2 years on average, while a girl baby could expect to live an average of 81.0 years.

These data differ by the race or ethnicity of the infant's mother, as shown in figure 2.1. Infants born to white mothers can expect to live several years longer on average than infants born to black mothers. The longest life expectancy of all these groups, however, is for infants born to Hispanic mothers.

We should note that life expectancy is reported separately for boys and for girls, as girls live several years longer than boys on average. Part of the gender difference in life expectancy can be explained by the hormonal differences that are a consequence of having either one X chromosome and one Y chromosome (male sex) or two X chromosomes (female sex). An additional part of the difference can be explained by differing patterns of behavior that develop during adolescence and early adulthood. For example, in 2010 the age-adjusted death rate (per 100,000 population) from motor vehicle accidents was 16.2 for males and 6.5 for females. If we look specifically at the motor vehicle death rate for those between 15 and 24 years of age, we see that the rate for men was 23.1, while that for women was 9.9 (CDCP 2013b). If instead we look at deaths from narcotic drug overdoses for those between 25 and 34 years of age, we see a male death rate of 25.0 and a female death rate

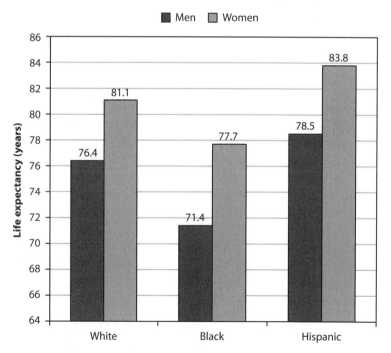

FIGURE 2.1. Life Expectancy at Birth in the United States by Gender and Race/Ethnicity, 2010. Data from US Centers for Disease Control and Prevention.

of 11.9 (CDCP 2013a). These gender-based differences in death rates among young adults have little to do with X versus Y chromosomes and everything to do with gender-based differences in behavior.

Infant mortality as a consequence of maternal behavior

An important contributor to observed differences in life expectancy at birth is the rate at which infants die before they reach the age of one year. Infant mortality rates are reported as deaths per 1,000 live births. As chromosome-based sex differences have little impact on the chances of death before age one, infant mortality rates usually are not reported based on the sex of the baby. More typically, they are reported based on the demographic characteristics of the mother.

In 2010 in the United States, the overall infant mortality rate was 6.1 (CDCP 2013c). This rate varied substantially based on the race and ethnicity of the mother. The infant mortality rate for infants born to white mothers was 5.2, while that for black mothers was 11.6—a black/white mortality ratio of 2.2:1. While overall infant mortality rates dropped substantially between 1950 and 2010 for both white and black infants, the ratio has actually widened. In 1950, the black/white ratio was 1.6:1.

To what extent do racial differences in infant mortality reflect underlying differences in maternal behavior? David and Collins (1997) addressed this issue in a study of the factors contributing to an increased incidence of infants born to black mothers in Illinois being born at a low birth weight—one of the principal risk factors for infant death. They identified a series of factors that put a mother at increased risk of having an infant with low birth weight. Principal among these were giving birth before age 20, being unmarried at the time of birth, never having finished high school, and being late in obtaining prenatal care. Compared to white mothers in Illinois who were born in the United States, black mothers in Illinois who were born in the United States had substantially higher rates of all these behavioral risk factors. Of note, the authors also found that black mothers who had been born in Africa but had subsequently moved to Illinois had behavioral risk profiles that were largely comparable to those of the white mothers as well as rates of low birth weight comparable to those of white mothers.

Sparks (2009) undertook a similar study, comparing mothers of different racial groups in the factors associated with an increased risk of giving birth prematurely—also a major risk factor for infant death. As with the study by David and Collins, Sparks found that behavioral differences on the part of the mother, rather than the mother's race or ethnicity, were the principal factors associated with premature birth. Principal among these at-risk behaviors were giving birth before age 20, not finishing high school, being unmarried at the time of birth, and gaining excess weight during pregnancy. Based on these findings, the author concluded "that pregnancy related behaviors are most important in offering potential explanations into the racial/ethnic disparity observed in preterm births" (p. 1674).

The CDCP has identified an additional risk factor associated with adverse infant outcomes. "Smoking during pregnancy causes additional health problems, including premature birth (being born too early), certain birth defects, and infant death." A federal publication from 2001 compared smoking rates among pregnant women and found that the highest rates were among Native American mothers and white mothers (Mathews 2001). In 1999, 20 percent of Native American and 15.7 percent of white mothers smoked during pregnancy, as compared to 9.1 percent of black mothers and 3.7 percent of Hispanic mothers. For both Native American and white mothers, the highest rates of smoking during pregnancy were found in women age 18-19. It seems clear that a woman's behaviors before becoming pregnant as well as during pregnancy are a major contributor to the risk of infant death and other adverse outcomes.

Life expectancy at age 25

Those who reach their 25th birthday no longer have to worry about the factors that cause death during infancy and childhood. These young adults are, however, affected by the choices they have made and the behaviors they have adopted in the process of reaching adulthood. It is valuable to see how many additional years, on average, 25-year-old men and women can expect to live and then to ask how differences in life expectancy might be associated with earlier patterns of behavior.

In 2011, the federal government reported on life expectancy for those turning 25 in 2006 (CDCP 2011). Once again, they reported data separately for men and women, also separating each gender into groups based on the highest level of education they had completed by the time they were 25. The results are shown in figure 2.2.

Once again we see a consistently greater life expectancy for women than for men at a comparable level of education. We also see another consistent pattern: the higher the level of education one has completed by age 25, the longer one can expect to live beyond age 25. Approaching one's investment in his or her education as an important form of behavior, we can see a powerful influence of the behaviors one adopts during the school years on one's subsequent well-being, using length of life as our measure of well-being.

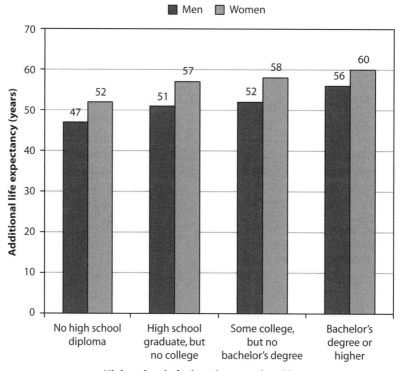

FIGURE 2.2. Life Expectancy in the United States at Age 25, by Gender and Highest Level of Education, 2006. Data from US Centers for Disease Control and Prevention, 2011.

Life expectancy at 65

Given the clear differences in life expectancy at age 25, it is valuable to examine what factors might affect one's life expectancy at an older age. Using data from federal databases for the year 2008, Olshansky and colleagues (2012) calculated the life expectancy for various age groups, broken down by gender, educational attainment, race, and ethnicity. Figure 2.3 shows life expectancy for these groups at age 65. For all the groups shown, we see a similar pattern of growing life expectancy for those with progressively higher levels of education. Since at age 65 these individuals will largely have completed their education decades earlier, we see the continuing effect of educational choices made decades earlier—typically in the adolescent years. While the magnitude of the disparity

at age 65 between those with the lowest levels of education and those with the highest levels has been reduced somewhat from its level at age 25, the disparity nonetheless continues to exist for all groups studied. Educational attainment as a form of behavior exhibited in childhood, adolescence, and early adulthood has continuing associations with well-being throughout the life course.

Since educational attainment is such a powerful predictor of life expectancy for all these gender and racial/ethnic groups, it seems pertinent to ask how the groups differ by average levels of educational attainment. The US Census Bureau (2012) reports educational attainment for different age groups and different racial and ethnic groups. Figure 2.4 shows the highest level of educational attainment of 65-year-olds in the United States in 2012. Focusing on the two highest levels

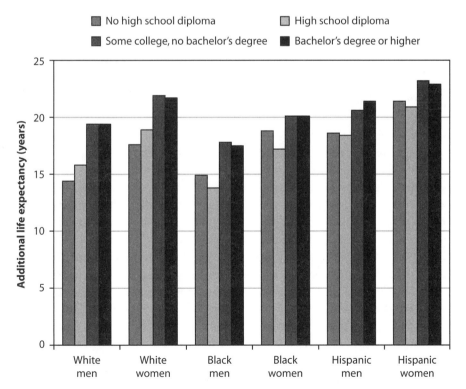

FIGURE 2.3. Life Expectancy in the United States at Age 65 by Gender, Race/Ethnicity, and Educational Attainment, 2008. Data from Olshansky et al. 2012.

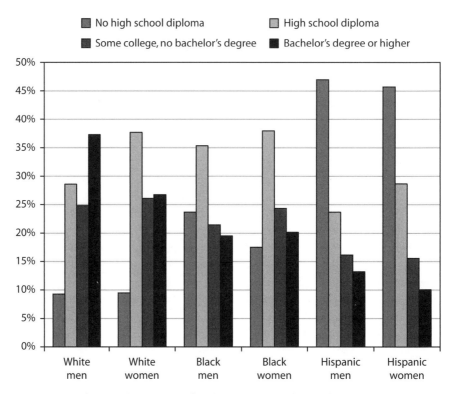

FIGURE 2.4. Educational Attainment for Those Age 65–69, by Gender and Race/Ethnicity, United States, 2012. Data from US Census Bureau.

shown—having completed some college, and having completed a bachelor's degree or higher—we see a higher educational level for white 65-year-olds than for black 65-year-olds, with Hispanics having the lowest level. While these racial and ethnic differences are substantial, we see only small differences by gender within each racial/ethnic group.

The data on life expectancy at birth and at age 65 in the United States are more meaningful when they are placed in a broader context. The Organisation for Economic Co-operation and Development (OECD) tracks and reports a range of health data on its 34 member states (OECD 2013). When we compare the United States to all 34 members of the OECD, including newer members from former Eastern bloc countries, we find that, in 2011, we ranked 22nd in life expectancy at age 65 for males and 25th for females.

Although we spend far more of our national budget on health care than any of these industrialized countries, the overall well-being of our population, measured as life expectancy, ranks toward the bottom. This brings up the question of what factors explain our relatively poor standing when compared to other countries.

Since 1991 the World Health Organization (WHO) has conducted a series of studies evaluating what they refer to as the Global Burden of Disease. Murray and Lopez (2013) reported on the findings of the report published by the WHO in 2010. The top six causes of death in the United States included ischemic heart disease, stroke, cancer of the lung and respiratory tract, dementia, chronic obstructive lung disease (a.k.a. emphysema), and diabetes.

Murray and his colleagues on the US Burden of Disease group that collaborated in the WHO report have published detailed data about the principal causes of death in the United States, the years of life lost to premature deaths that were potentially preventable, and the US ranking on these indices (Murray et al. 2013). They reported that the years of life lost in the United States to preventable deaths placed us 28th among OECD countries when ranking countries from the lowest to the highest preventable death rates. Only Poland, Slovakia, Estonia, Hungary, Mexico, and Turkey had higher rates of preventable deaths.

Murray and colleagues assessed the principal risk factors leading to this high rate of premature, preventable deaths in the United States. The top six factors, in order of their association with premature death, were diet, tobacco use, high blood pressure, high body mass index (i.e., obesity), physical inactivity, and elevated blood sugar due to diabetes. The researchers identified specific dietary risks associated with premature deaths, in particular "diets low in fruits, low in nuts and seeds, high in sodium [salt], high in processed meats, low in vegetables, and high in *trans* fats" (p. 596). If, as described in chapter 1, behavior is a response to our perception and interpretation of external stimuli, it would appear that these dietary patterns reflect unhealthy behaviors. Do these dietary patterns reflect a conscious choice of less healthy food over more healthy alternatives? The answer depends on the extent to which behavior reflects conscious choice rather than learned patterns of response. We explore these issues in more depth in later chapters.

Mokdad and colleagues (2004) undertook a similar study of the causes of death in the United States, examining the extent to which these were associated with behaviors that might be preventable. They analyzed the leading causes of death in 2000 in the United States and found that heart disease, cancer, cerebrovascular disease such as stroke, and chronic lung disease accounted for 65 percent of all deaths. When they used epidemiological data to evaluate the association between certain behaviors and the likelihood of death, they determined that the actual causes of death, rather than the specific diseases leading to death, were health behaviors that increased the likelihood or severity of the disease. From this analysis they were able to determine that tobacco use and poor diet together accounted directly for 33 percent of all deaths and 69 percent of potentially preventable deaths.

The Institute of Medicine of the National Academy of Sciences convened a national workshop to further explore the analyses of Mokdad and colleagues. The intent of the workshop was to "enrich understanding of the contribution of lifestyle-related factors to preventable death and . . . the role of preventable death as a driving force in public health" (Institute of Medicine 2005, p. 2). At the conclusion of the workshop, participants concurred on the importance of behavioral factors in causing premature death and as a consequence reducing life expectancy in the United States. They also went a step further, suggesting that the public health professionals and those responsible for setting policy "focus on lifestyle-related risks as a collective problem" and that they "reframe the debate to focus on the impact of proposed interventions rather than risk factors" (p. 50).

This growing awareness of the policy implications of health-related behaviors and their consequence, and the need to intervene to prevent these behaviors before they cause harm, underscore the importance of understanding how patterns of human behavior develop. We are again confronted by the issue of whether behaviors such as smoking, diet, and exercise represent conscious choices or learned patterns of response. Recall from figure 1.1 that the level of education an individual attains is highly predictive of his or her likelihood of becoming a smoker as an adult. Similarly, data from the CDCP have identified a significant inverse association between level of education and prevalence of obesity among women, with less of an association among men (Ogden et al. 2010). Shaw

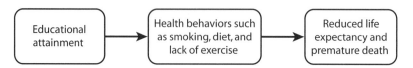

FIGURE 2.5. Educational Attainment, Health Risk Behaviors, and Preventable Deaths in the United States

and Spokane (2008) have also identified a direct association between level of educational attainment and level of physical activity as an adult, with the differences in exercise between those with lower levels of education and those with higher levels widening over time after about age 55. Thus, in understanding the causes of premature mortality in the United States, it appears that a stepwise model of associations is most appropriate, as illustrated in figure 2.5.

Much of the cause of the poor levels of life expectancy relative to other developed countries is attributable to three principal behaviors: smoking, diet, and exercise. In turn, one's level of these behaviors as an adult is consistently associated with the level of education one has attained by early adulthood. The relatively low life expectancy at birth of infants born in the United States is reflected in the strong subsequent association between educational attainment at age 25 and additional life expectancy, as illustrated in figure 2.2. Educational attainment seems to reflect a form of behavior that is closely associated with other behaviors exhibited throughout the life course. If behavior is a response to the perception and interpretation of stimuli from the environment, this raises the pressing question of what stimuli children and adolescents are responding to when they adopt their own behavioral approaches to school and other educational opportunities.

Physical well-being beyond life expectancy

So far, we have been looking at physical well-being primarily in terms of life expectancy and rates of mortality. Another approach to physical well-being considers the quality of the life experience. Living ten years free of disabilities can be a profoundly different experience than living those same ten years with one or more disabilities that impair one's level of activity and social interaction.

The World Health Organization has been working since 1990 to develop a standardized metric that reflects both the expected length of life within a population group as well as the level of disability experienced by that group. In 1994, Murray reported on those efforts with a technical description of a new metric, the "disability-adjusted life year," often referred to as the DALY. Murray identified two principles on which he based the development of this metric:

- any measure of health outcome should include consideration of the loss of welfare caused by a disability; and
- using time as a measure of the burden of disease should include both this loss of welfare as well as time lost to premature mortality.

In order to combine the loss of welfare with the premature loss of life, Murray identified six different levels of disability, described in table 2.1. He assigned each of these a numerical weight, based on the severity of the impact of the disability, with weights varying from 0.096 to 0.920. By multiplying the years a person lives with a disability by the decimal weight of the level of disability experienced, it is possible to calculate the years of disability-free life lost as a consequence of the disability. For example, living

TABLE 2.1. Definition and Weighting of Levels of Disability Used to Calculate Disability-Adjusted Life Years

Disability class	Disability weight	Description of disability
1	.096	Limited ability to perform at least one activity in one of the following areas: recreation, education, procreation, or occupation
2	.220	Limited ability to perform most activities in one of the following areas: recreation, education, procreation, or occupation
3	.400	Limited ability to perform activities in two or more of the following areas: recreation, education, procreation, or occupation
4	.600	Limited ability to perform most activities in all of the following areas: recreation, education, procreation, or occupation
5	.810	Needs assistance with instrumental activities of daily living such as meal preparation, shopping, or housework
6	.920	Needs assistance with activities of daily living such as eating, personal hygiene, or toilet use

Source: Murray 2010.

10 years with a Class 4 disability, which carries a weight of 0.600, would mean the loss of 6 of those 10 years, referred to as the loss of 6 DALYs. Thus, calculating the years of life lost to potentially preventable causes, DALYs account both for the loss due to disability and the loss due to premature death.

In 2012, Murray et al. reported the findings of the Global Burden of Disease (GBD) study from 2010, a major international undertaking involving close to 500 researchers from 50 countries, representing more than 300 academic and research institutions. Extending work done in an initial GBD study published in 1990, Murray described the 2010 GBD as "The only comprehensive effort to date to estimate summary measures of population health for the world, by cause." Consistent with his 1994 work, "For a summary measure of population health, the GBD study uses disability-adjusted life years (DALYs), which are the sum of years of life lost due to premature mortality (YLL) and years lived with disability (YLD)." (p. 2198)

One of the principal findings of the study was the "relatively small changes in the number of DALYs" lost globally between 1990 and 2010, "because the increase in the global population has been largely balanced by a decrease in the age-sex-specific DALY rates" (p. 2215). They also found a substantial shift from loss due to premature death to loss due to increasing rates of disability from mental illness and other forms of chronic illness.

As part of this global focus on gaining a better understanding of population health, the CDCP has developed a metric called "active life expectancy," described as the "expected years free of chronic condition-induced activity limitations" (Molla and Madans 2010, p. 2). Using this metric, the authors assessed changes in the United States between 2000 and 2006 in active life expectancy and found that it increased for all population groups with the exception of those age 85 or older. They did note that, while active life expectancy at ages 25, 45, and 65 had increased for both blacks and whites, the black/white disparity remained largely unchanged at all ages.

In 2013 Molla published an updated assessment of health in the United States as part of a broader Health Disparities and Inequalities Report published by the CDCP (Meyer et al. 2013). He again documented continuing improvements in expected years of life free of activity limitations but noted continuing disparities between blacks and whites in these measures. This finding is part of the more general identification by the report of "persistent disparities between some population groups in health outcomes, access to health care, adoption of health promoting behaviors, and exposure to health-promoting environments" (Meyer et al. 2013, p. 184).

An earlier report by the CDCP (2008a) looked specifically at which forms of disability most affected healthy life expectancy and examined the behavioral factors associated with those disabilities. In this analysis, it differentiated between "basic actions difficulty," described as "limitations or difficulties in movement and sensory, emotional, or mental functioning that are associated with some health problem," and "complex activity limitation," described as "limitations or restrictions in a person's ability to participate fully in social role activities such as working or maintaining a household" (p. 5).

For the period 2001–2005, the prevalence of basic actions difficulty among adults aged 18 or older was 29.5 percent while the prevalence of complex activity limitations was 14.3 percent. Approximately one-third of both types of limitations were found in adults aged 65 years or older, with the balance in those younger than 65. Looking at the association between education and level of disability, the highest rates of disability were seen in those who either had not finished high school or who had graduated from high school but not pursued further education, with the lowest rates among those who had graduated from college.

The report went on to examine the association between certain behavioral risk factors and the level of disability experienced. Consistent with the associations described above between behavior and life expectancy, the report identified clear associations between behavior and disability, with:

- "adults with disabilities less likely to be of healthy weight and more likely to be obese than adults without disability" (p. 34);
- "adults with disabilities more likely to be current smokers than adults with no disability" (p. 37); and
- "adults with all the types of disability measured here less likely to participate in regular leisure-time physical activity than adults with no disability" (p. 38).

Muennig et al. (2010) reported a similar analysis in which they examined the association between certain behaviors, quality of life, and length of life using a measure referred to as the "quality-adjusted life year" (QALY), calculated in a manner quite similar to the DALY. As shown in table 2.2, they found that living with an income less than twice the federal poverty level and never having finished high school were the strongest demographic predictors of reduced life expectancy measured in QALYs, while smoking and obesity were the principal behavioral factors.

Rather than using broad demographic data to quantify the effects of behaviors and demographic characteristics on the length of life adjusted for quality of life, a number of researchers have used a far simpler approach to assessing the health status of individuals. They ask individuals how they would describe their own health, using the categories of excellent, very good, good, fair, or poor. It turns out that this simple measure can provide valuable and accurate information about an individual's overall health.

TABLE 2.2. Mean Quality-Adjusted Life Years (QALYs) Lost between Ages 18 and 85 in Association with Behaviors and Demographic Characteristics

Risk factor	QALYs lost
Smoking	6.6
Obesity	4.2
Binge drinking	1.2
Education (not finishing high school as compared to high school graduation or more)	5.1
Poverty (income less than twice the federal poverty level, after adjusting for education)	6.4
Race (black as compared to white, after adjusting for education)	1.7

Source: Muennig et al. 2010.

This was the measure used by Lee et al. (2007) in their study of more than 16,000 adults aged 50 or greater. In 1998 they evaluated the self-rated health of each subject using this scale, and then they followed the subjects for four years to measure the age-adjusted death rate of different racial groups. For both black and white subjects, there was a consistent, stepwise association between each category of self-rated health and the subsequent death rate, with the largest increments found for those reporting fair or poor health. The authors then divided health reports into two categories: good (reported as excellent, very good, or good) and poor (reported as fair or poor). Using multivariate analysis to control for factors such as gender, race, and education, they found consistent associations between self-rated health and the subsequent risk of death in all age groups, with the exception of those age 80 or older.

The CDCP (2008b) also assessed the extent to which self-rated health is associated with one's level of disability. In a study of a range of racial and ethnic groups, they reported that "adults with a disability were less likely to report excellent or very good health (27.2 percent versus 60.2 percent; $p<0.01$) and more likely to report fair or poor health (40.3 percent versus 9.9 percent; $p<0.01$)" (p. 1070). They also found that Hispanics and American Indian/Alaska Natives reported the highest rates of fair or poor health, with whites and Asians reporting the lowest.

Zajacova et al. (2012) evaluated the association between the level of educational attainment and self-rated health status, using data gathered as part of a nationally representative study of more than 178,000 working-age adults in the United States. Using the same five-category measure of self-rated health, they found that "health is strongly related to education for all levels of educational attainment. Each additional credential or educational level is associated with significantly better health, from high school graduation all the way up through the professional and doctoral degrees" (p. 55). In looking for other factors that would affect this education/health gradient, they found two with significant associations: economic indicators (employment status and family income) and health behaviors (smoking, obesity, and alcohol use).

Leopold and Engelhardt (2013) conducted a similar study using data from a survey of nearly 15,000 adults between the ages of 50 and 80 living in a range of countries in Europe. They found higher levels of self-rated health and lower levels of chronic diseases in those with higher levels of education.

Bauldry et al. (2012) looked at the other end of the age spectrum in their study of the self-rated health status of children and adolescents in the United States, initially surveyed when they were between the ages of 11 and 19 and then followed into their twenties and early thirties. When the subjects were in their early teens, the principal predictors of lower self-rated health were lower family socioeconomic position and stressful family situations. As the subjects grew into later adolescence and early adulthood, these background factors became less important, and the health behaviors of the subjects themselves become more predictive. Principal among the behaviors associated with lower health status were obesity, alcohol use, smoking, and physical inactivity.

Before ending our discussion of self-rated health status, we should acknowledge one caveat: one's perception of his or her health status on the scales utilized in these studies does not necessarily equate with one's perception of his or her overall quality of life. Individuals with substantial levels of disability may nonetheless perceive their quality of life as indistinguishable from others who do not experience those disabilities. This principle has been illustrated in work by Saigal et al. (2006), in their study of young adults who were born extremely prematurely at a time when such infants had a substantial probability of experiencing lifelong physical or emotional impairments as a consequence of their prematurity.

Saigal followed 140 subjects who were born in the period 1977-1982 weighing between 500 and 1,000 grams—a category referred to as extremely low birth weight (ELBW). She followed these subjects into their early twenties and compared them to a comparable group of young adults who had been born during the same time period at a normal birth weight (NBW) of greater than 2,500 grams. For both groups she assessed their self-rated health status and, on a separate scale, their self-rated overall quality of life. She identified major differences in self-reported health status, with the ELBW subjects reporting significantly higher rates of physical and emotional impairment in a number of areas. However, when compared on self-rated quality of life, there were no significant differences between the two groups, leading Dr. Saigal to caution against the "prevailing perception among individuals without disabilities ... that a good

quality of life is not possible, or at least is unlikely, when serious ill health or disability is present" (p. 1144). Quite the contrary, Saigal points out, "most ELBW subjects have made remarkable adjustments in many aspects of their lives by the time they reach young adulthood. It is therefore not surprising that their [health-related quality of life] is no different from that of their NBW peers" (p. 1147). We should keep this principle in mind when, in later chapters, we discuss how adolescents and young adults can adopt differing psychological perspectives about how they perceive themselves and their roles in life.

Social well-being

Individuals rarely live in isolation from others. Children interact with their families and peers; adults interact with their families, neighbors, peers, and communities. A key aspect of human well-being is the extent and the quality of these social interactions.

Kawachi (1999) has described this concept as "social capital," which he describes as referring "to those features of social relationships—such as levels of interpersonal trust and norms of reciprocity and mutual aid—that facilitate collective action for mutual benefit" (p. 120). He suggests that experiencing enhanced social capital is associated with a number of positive outcomes, including reduced rates of juvenile delinquency and crime, enhanced education, and increased economic opportunity.

Kawachi and Berkman (2000) contrast the concept of social networks with social capital: "Social networks are a characteristic that can (and most often have been) be measured at the individual level, whereas social capital should be properly considered a characteristic of the collective (neighbourhood, community, society) to which the individual belongs" (p. 176). As we will see, there is evidence that both forms of social interaction—one's own social networks and the broader social capital of one's community—enhance well-being.

Social networks

Sociologists and other social and behavioral scientists have become increasingly interested in the types of social connections individuals make with others and how those connections affect their well-being. The characteristics of a social network reflect the types of people an individual interacts with (family, friends, neighbors, coworkers, etc.), the quality of the relationship (close, trusting, etc.), and the frequency with which one interacts with those in her or his network.

The value of social networks for well-being has been shown in a variety of contexts. For example, Cohen et al. (1997) evaluated the factors affecting the chances an otherwise healthy individual would come down with a cold when exposed to a known dose of cold virus in a controlled laboratory setting. After controlling for a range of other factors, they found that those subjects with the greatest social network diversity were less likely to come down with a cold after exposure to the virus, suggesting that the strength of one's social networks enhances the ability to fight off a cold virus.

In a rather different context, Semenza et al. (1996) looked at the association of an individual's social networks and the chance they would have died in the intense heat wave that struck Chicago in 1995, in which temperatures remained above 100 degrees for several days running. Among the other factors associated with an increased chance of death, the authors found that living alone and having few regular social contacts increased the chances of death.

Social networks have been shown to be of particular value to older adults. Crooks et al. (2008) followed a sample of about 2,249 women age 78 or older, none of whom showed signs of dementia at the initial evaluation. Four years after their initial assessment, 209 of the women had died and 432 had dropped out of the study. Of the 1,608 subjects remaining, 268 (17%) exhibited evidence of dementia using a standardized assessment tool. Study participants with larger social networks showed a significantly reduced risk of dementia. More regular contact with other people one is familiar with appears to provide a protective effect on continued cognitive ability among the elderly.

White et al. (2009) studied a randomly selected sample of about 3,500 adults age 60 and over who had participated in a national survey of health status. Subjects were asked to describe their health status using the five-step excellent-poor scale described above. The authors of this study collapsed these responses into three categories: poor, fair/good, and very good/excellent. They then looked at the association between the strength of the emotional support these individuals received from their social networks and their self-rated health using this scale, after statistically controlling for age, race, gender, and educational attainment. Consistent with the study by Crooks et al., this study found that stronger support provided by one's social network was significantly associated with better self-reported health status.

These results raise the question as to whether social networks can enhance the emotional well-being of younger adults as well. A team of social science researchers who focus on the dynamics of social networks and their association with well-being have published a series of studies examining this question. They use data gathered from the Framingham Heart Study, one of the longest running longitudinal studies of adult health status in the United States. From these analyses they were able to identify the following associations:

- "Depression depends on how connected individuals are and where they are located in social networks," with the level of depression experienced by individuals correlated with the level of depression in one's friends and neighbors (Rosenquist et al. 2011, p. 280).
- "Loneliness not only spreads from person to person within a social network but it also

reduces the ties of these individuals to others within the network. As a result loneliness is found in clusters within social networks" (Cacioppo et al. 2009, p. 986).

- "People who are surrounded by many happy people and those who are central in the network are more likely to become happy in the future . . . People's happiness depends on the happiness of others with whom they are connected" (Fowler and Christakis 2008, p. 1).

It thus appears that the strength of one's relations to others is associated with well-being in a variety of ways, including physical health status, cognitive ability, and emotional well-being. These findings raise some interesting questions. Does participation in social networks constitute a form of behavior analogous to smoking, diet, and exercise? Are there certain personality characteristics that make it easier or more difficult for an individual to participate actively in social networks? We return to this issue in chapter 7, when we discuss various theories of personality development.

Social capital, as distinct from social networks

The concept of social capital is seen as reflecting a different level of social interaction than one's personal social networks. While networks reflect the direct interactions between groups of individuals, social capital reflects qualities that develop in the broader social environment in which one lives or works. As described above, social capital reflects concepts such as the level of trust one perceives in his or her community and the sense that if we help others around us, they will reciprocate by helping us should we need it.

Murayama et al. (2012) conducted a comprehensive review of published studies of the association between social capital and health. They indicated that the various studies tended to focus on two aspects of social capital. The first, which they refer to as social cohesion, "represents resources available to members of tightly knit communities." The second, which seems closer to the concept of social networks discussed above, refers to "resources that are embedded within an individual's social networks" (p. 179). Some of the studies focused on residential communities, while others reported on the workplace. The review found consistent associations between social capital and mortality rates, self-rated health status, health-related behaviors, and mental depression, leading the authors to conclude that both forms of social capital "appear to have positive effects on health outcomes" (p. 184).

A number of authors have reported similar studies conducted in European countries of the associations between social capital and health, with similar results (Mohnen et al. 2011; Kim et al. 2011). Nieminen et al. (2013) studied the association of social capital, health behaviors (smoking, alcohol use, diet, exercise), and overall health. They reported that "Irrespective of their social status, people with higher levels of social capital . . . engage in healthier behaviors and feel healthier both physically and psychologically" (p. 1).

This issue—whether there is a link between the level of social inequality in a community and the association between social capital and health within that community—was studied by De Clercq et al. (2012) in their study of communities in Belgium. They reported three main conclusions: (1) that an individual's economic affluence was positively associated with perceived health and well-being; (2) that the social capital of one's community had a stronger association with individual health than social capital measured at the level of the individual; and (3) while communities with higher levels of economic inequality tended to have worse health status, stronger social capital narrowed these economic differences substantially.

These results raise an important issue. How do levels of economic capital and social capital compare in their associations with well-being? Ahnquist et al. (2012) studied this question in a survey of more than 50,000 individuals in Sweden between the ages of 18 and 84. They measured health status as both self-rated health and psychological health. Both lower economic capital and lower social capital were significantly associated with worse health status, with the worst health present in those who experience low levels of both forms of capital. We will discuss the effects of social capital and cultural capital again in chapter 5 when we consider the work of Pierre Bourdieu.

Social inequality can affect well-being adversely in a number of ways. That inequality can be economic in nature, social in nature, or both simultaneously. Individual behavior over the life course plays a substantial role in affecting both one's economic circumstances and one's social circumstances, and in turn the level of inequality one experiences. There are, of course, broader social forces that are not the result of individual behaviors yet nonetheless impact levels of inequality within a society. In the next chapter we will look at the many ways in which inequality, behavior, and well-being seem to be inextricably linked.

Summary

Human well-being is experienced in a variety of ways. Mortality rates and associated levels of life expectancy are common measures used to compare societies and social groups. Both are clearly associated with certain behaviors, principal among them smoking, diet, exercise, and excessive alcohol use. These behaviors in turn are closely associated with the level of education one has attained by early adulthood.

Well-being, though, is a broader concept than mortality rates alone. One's well-being can be powerfully affected by the level of disability experienced over time and by the extent to which that disability affects one's quality of life. Beyond physical impairments, psychological impairments such as depression can also affect well-being. Often simply asking individuals to rate their own health status on a five-step scale from "excellent" to "poor" will provide accurate and useful information about these aspects of well-being. Once again, we see consistent associations between individual health behaviors and these aspects of well-being. Finally, we have seen associations between an individual's social circumstances, approached either as the nature of her or his own social networks or as the level of social cohesion within one's broader community, and well-being assessed in a number of ways.

How should we view the role of education in these relationships? Greater educational attainment is association with fewer unhealthy behaviors and with enhanced well-being in a range of contexts. Is educational attainment a form of behavior that is analogous to smoking and diet? We certainly know that greater educational attainment usually leads to greater economic well-being, which brings with it various forms of enhanced well-being. We also know, however, that growing up in circumstances of economic and social inequality is often associated with lower levels of educational attainment. This again raises the question of the role of social and economic inequality in affecting well-being, the focus of the next chapter.

REFERENCES

Ahnquist, J., Wamala, S. P., & Lindstrom, M. 2012. Social determinants of health—A question of social or economic capital? Interaction effects of socioeconomic factors on health outcomes. Social Science and Medicine 74(6): 930–39.

Bauldry, S., Shanahan, M. J., Boardman, J. D., Miech, R. A., & Macmillan, R. 2012. A life course model of self-rated health through adolescence and young adulthood. Social Science and Medicine 75(7): 1311–20.

Cacioppo, J. T., Fowler, J. H., & Christakis, N. A. 2009. Alone in the crowd: The structure and spread of loneliness in a large social network. Journal of Personality and Social Psychology 97(6): 977–91.

Centers for Disease Control and Prevention, US Department of Health and Human Services. 2008a. Disability and health in the United States, 2001-2005. DHHS Publication No. (PHS) 2008-1035, available at www.cdc.gov/nchs/data/misc/disability2001-2005.pdf, accessed 12/19/13.

———. 2008b. Racial/ethnic differences in self-rated health status among adults with and without disabilities—United States, 2004-2006. Morbidity and Mortality Weekly Report 57(39): 1069-73.

———. 2011. Life expectancy at age 25, by sex and education level: United States, 1996 and 2006, available at www.cdc.gov/nchs/data/hus/2011/fig32.pdf, accessed 11/26/13.

———. 2013a. Death rates for drug poisoning and drug poisoning involving opioid analgesics, by sex, age, race, and Hispanic origin: United States, selected years 1999-2010, available at www.cdc.gov/nchs/data/hus/2012/032.pdf, accessed 11/26/13.

———. 2013b. Death rates for motor vehicle-related injuries, by sex, race, Hispanic origin, and age: United States, selected years 1950-2010, available at www.cdc.gov/nchs/data/hus/2012/033.pdf, accessed 11/26/13.

———. 2013c. Infant mortality rates, fetal mortality rates, and perinatal mortality rates, by race: United States, selected years 1950-2010, available at www.cdc.gov/nchs/data/hus/2012/013.pdf, accessed 11/26/13.

———. 2013d. Life expectancy at birth, at age 65, and at age 75, by sex, race, and Hispanic origin: United States, selected years 1900-2010, available at www.cdc.gov/nchs/data/hus/2012/018.pdf, accessed 11/26/13.

———. How does smoking during pregnancy harm my health and my baby? Available at www.cdc.gov/reproductivehealth/TobaccoUsePregnancy/index.htm, accessed 11/26/13.

———. Well-being concepts, available at www.cdc.gov/hrqol/wellbeing.htm#three, accessed 11/25/13.

Cohen, S., Doyle, W. J., Skoner, D. P., Rabin, B. S., & Gwaltney, J. M. 1997. Social ties and susceptibility to the common cold. JAMA 277: 1940-44.

Crooks, V. C., Lubben, J., Petitti, D. B., Little, D., & Chiu, V. 2008. Social network, cognitive function, and dementia incidence among elderly women. American Journal of Public Health 98(7): 1221-27.

David, R. J., & Collins, J. W. 1997. Differing birth weight among infants of U.S.-born blacks, African-born blacks, and U.S.-born whites. New England Journal of Medicine 337: 1209-14.

De Clercq, B., Vyncke, V., Hublet, A., et al. 2012. Social capital and social inequality in adolescents' health in 601 Flemish communities: A multilevel analysis. Social Science and Medicine 74(2): 202-10.

Fowler, J. H., & Christakis, N. A. 2008. Dynamic spread of happiness in a large social network: Longitudinal analysis over 20 years in the Framingham Heart Study. BMJ 337: a2338.

Institute of Medicine. Planning Committee on Estimating the Contributions of Lifestyle-Related Factors to Preventable Death; Board on Population Health and Public Health Practice. 2005. Estimating the contributions of lifestyle-related factors to preventable death: A workshop summary. www.nap.edu/catalog.php?Record_id=11323, accessed 11/29/13.

Kawachi, I. 1999. Social capital and community effects on population and individual death. Annals of the New York Academy of Sciences 896: 120-30.

Kawachi, I., & Berkman, L. 2000. Social cohesion, social capital, and health. In Berkman, L., and Kawachi, I., ed. Social Epidemiology, 174-90. New York: Oxford University Press.

Kim, D., Baum, C. F., Ganz, M. L., Subramanian, S. V., & Kawachi, I. 2011. The contextual effects of social capital on health: A cross-national instrumental variable analysis. Social Science and Medicine 73(12): 1689-97.

Lee, A. S., Moody-Ayers, S. Y., Landefeld, C. S., et al. 2007. The relationship between self-rated health and mortality in older black and white Americans. Journal of the American Geriatrics Society 55(10): 1624-29.

Leopold, L. , & Engelhardt, H. 2013. Education and physical health trajectories in old age. Evidence from the Survey of Health, Ageing and Retirement in Europe (SHARE). International Journal of Public Health 58(1): 23-31.

Mathews, T. J. 2001. Smoking during pregnancy in the 1990s. National Vital Statistics Report 49(7), available at www.cdc.gov/nchs/data/nvsr/nvsr49/nvsr49_07.pdf, accessed 11/26/13.

Meyer, P. A., Yoon, P. W., & Kaufmann, R. B. 2013. CDC health disparities and inequalities report—United States, 2013. Morbidity and Mortality Weekly Report 62(3): 1-187.

Mohnen, S. M., Groenewegen, P. P., Völker, B., & Flap, H. 2011. Neighborhood social capital and individual health. Social Science and Medicine 72(5): 660-67.

Mokdad, A. H., Marks, J. S., Stroup, D. F., & Gerberding, J. L. 2004. Actual causes of death in the United States, 2000. JAMA 291: 1238-45.

Molla, M. T. 2013. Expected years of life free of chronic condition-induced activity limitations—United States, 1999-2008. Morbidity and Mortality Weekly Report 62(3): 87-91.

Molla, M. T., & Madans, J. H. 2010. Life expectancy free of chronic condition-induced activity limitations among white and black Americans, 2000-2006. CDCP

Vital and Health Statistics Series 3, Number 34, available at www.cdc.gov/nchs/data/series/sr_03/sr03_034.pdf, accessed 12/18/13.

Muennig, P., Fiscella, K., Tancredi, D., & Franks, P. 2010. The relative health burden of selected social and behavioral risk factors in the United States: Implications for policy. American Journal of Public Health 100(9): 1758-64.

Murayama, H., Fujiwara, Y., & Kawachi, I. 2012. Social capital and health: A review of prospective multilevel studies. Journal of Epidemiology 22(3): 179-87.

Murray, C. J. L. 1994. Quantifying the burden of disease: The technical basis for disability-adjusted life years. Bulletin of the World Health Organization 72(3): 429-45.

Murray, C. J. L., & Lopez, A. D. 2013. Measuring the global burden of disease. New England Journal of Medicine 369: 448-57.

Murray, C. J. L., & US Burden of Disease Collaborators. 2013. The state of US health, 1990-2010: Burden of diseases, injuries, and risk factors. JAMA 310(6): 591-608.

Murray, C. J. L., Vos, T., Lozano, R., et al. 2012. Disability-adjusted life years (DALYs) for 291 diseases and injuries in 21 regions, 1990-2010: A systematic analysis for the Global Burden of Disease Study 2010. The Lancet 380: 2197-223.

Nieminen, T., Prättälä, R., Martelin, T., et al. 2013. Social capital, health behaviours and health: A population-based associational study. BMC Public Health 13: 613.

Ogden, C. L., Lamb, M. M., Carroll, M. D., & Flegal, K. M. 2010. Obesity and socioeconomic status in adults: United States, 2005-2008. NCHS Data Brief, Number 50, available at www.cdc.gov/nchs/data/databriefs/db50.htm, accessed 11/29/13.

Olshansky, S. J., Antonucci, T., Berkman, L., et al. 2012. Differences in life expectancy due to race and educational differences are widening, and many may not catch up. Health Affairs 31: 1803+Appendix.

Organisation for Economic Co-operation and Development. Health data 2013: Frequently requested data, available at www.oecd.org/health/health-systems/oecdhealthdata2013-frequentlyrequesteddata.htm, accessed 11/27/13.

Rosenquist, J. N., Fowler, J. H., & Christakis, N. A. 2011. Social network determinants of depression. Molecular Psychiatry 16(3): 273-81.

Saigal, S., Stoskopf, B., Pinelli, J., et al. 2006. Self-perceived health-related quality of life of former extremely low birth weight infants at young adulthood. Pediatrics 118(3): 1140-48.

Semenza, J. C., Rubin, C. H., Falter, K. H., et al. 1996. Heat-related deaths during the July 1995 heat wave in Chicago. New England Journal of Medicine 335: 84-90.

Shaw, B. A., & Spokane, L. S. 2008. Examining the association between education level and physical activity changes during early old age. Journal of Aging and Health 20: 767-87.

Sparks, P. J. 2009. Do biological, sociodemographic, and behavioral characteristics explain racial/ethnic disparities in preterm births? Social Science and Medicine 68: 1667-75.

US Census Bureau. Educational attainment in the United States: 2012, available at www.census.gov/hhes/socdemo/education/data/cps/2012/tables.html, accessed 11/27/13.

White, A. M., Philogene, G. S., Fine, L., & Sinha, S. 2009. Social support and self-reported health status of older adults in the United States. American Journal of Public Health 99(10): 1872-78.

World Health Organization. Global burden of disease, described at www.who.int/topics/global_burden_of_disease/en, accessed 11/29/13.

Zajacova, A., Hummer, R. A., & Rogers, R. G. 2012. Education and health among US working-age adults: A detailed portrait across the full educational attainment spectrum. Biodemography and Social Biology 58(1): 40-61.

CHAPTER 3

Inequality and Well-Being

Well-being as an adult is largely tied to a relatively small set of health-related behaviors. Whether looking at life expectancy, level of disability, or self-reported health status, we see that smoking, obesity, and patterns of diet and exercise consistently impact well-being adversely. We also see that educational attainment by the age of 25 is consistently associated with these behaviors, with those completing lower levels of education more often engaging in unhealthy behaviors and as a consequence experiencing reduced well-being throughout adulthood.

There is another, equally important aspect of differences in life expectancy that we should acknowledge and explore. As shown in figure 3.1, taken from Olshansky et al. (2012), there is clear evidence that those with lower levels of education completed by age 25 have a shorter life expectancy than those with a higher level. This association is a continuous one, through all levels of education shown. The second association illustrated by the figure is the clear racial and ethnic difference in life expectancy among the groups shown. At every level of educational attainment, and for both genders, black life expectancy is lower than white life expectancy, and white life expectancy is lower than Hispanic life expectancy.

Racial and ethnic inequality in health in association with educational inequality

Wong et al. (2002) examined the relative influence of race and educational attainment on black and white mortality rates. As described by the authors in introducing their study, "Mortality from all causes is higher for persons with fewer years of education and for blacks, but it is unknown which diseases contribute most to these disparities" (p. 1585). Using nationally representative data from the 1980s and 1990s, they compared mortality rates and the principal cause of death, first by comparing those

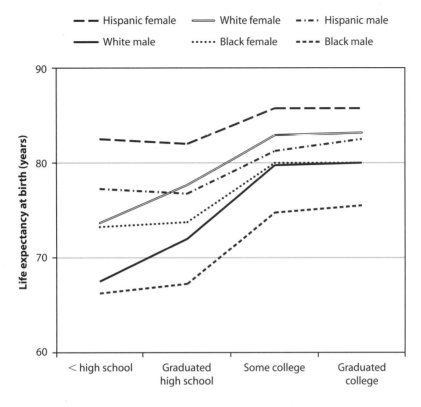

FIGURE 3.1. Life Expectancy at Birth, by Years of Education at Age 25, by Race and Sex, 2008. Data from Olshansky et al. 2012.

with lower education to those with higher education while controlling for age, gender, and race. They then repeated the analysis, comparing black adults with white adults while controlling for age, gender, and level of education. They found that differential rates of death due to cardiovascular disease such as heart attacks or strokes and death due to cancer explained most of the difference in both comparisons, with causes such as infections and other forms of lung disease playing a lesser role. They also found that the impact on mortality rates was greater for educational differences than it was for racial differences. In their discussion of these research results they emphasized two findings:

1. "The level of education and race each appear to have strong, independent effects that persist after controlling for the other" (p. 1591).

2. "A few conditions account for most of these disparities—smoking-related diseases in the case of mortality among persons with fewer years of education, and hypertension, HIV, diabetes mellitus, and trauma in the case of mortality among black persons" (p. 1585).

Researchers at the US Centers for Disease Control and Prevention (CDCP) reported the results of a similar analysis using data for 2010 (Kochanek et al. 2013). They noted that although overall life expectancy had increased steadily between 1970 and 2010, a substantial disparity between black and white life expectancy persisted throughout that time frame. In 2010, life expectancy in the United States was 4.7 years longer for white men than for black men and 3.3 years longer for white women than for black women. Researchers then asked which causes of death contributed most to this disparity. For men, the principal causes of the higher black mortality rate were heart disease, homicide, cancer, and stroke, while for women the principal causes were heart disease, cancer, diabetes, and stroke. As discussed in the previous chapter, these conditions are closely linked to behaviors such as smoking, diet, and exercise. It thus appears that inequality in life expectancy in the United States is linked both to education and to race independent of education.

If we look at levels of disability rather than rates of mortality, we see a similar pattern. In 2013 the CDCP published an updated *Health Disparities and Inequalities Report* that offered an assessment of current "health disparities and inequalities across a wide range of diseases, behavioral risk factors, environmental exposures, social determinants, and health-care access by sex, race and ethnicity, income, education, disability status and other social characteristics" (CDCP 2013). Using data for 2011, the report first noted that not having finished high school was the most consistent predictor of the outcomes it studied. Not surprisingly, those who did not complete high school were substantially more likely to be poor or near poor than those with higher levels of education. In addition, those who did not complete high school were substantially more likely to report a current disability. (These analyses adjusted for age differences among groups.)

The report then looked at race and ethnicity and found failure to complete high school occurring more commonly in three groups: black, Hispanic, and American Indian. Using these data, the report then calculated the expected years of life free of activity limitations due to

chronic conditions. In 2008, blacks in the United States could expect 5.9 fewer years of life without disability than whites. (This was actually a decrease in the black/white disparity from 1999, when blacks could expect 7.0 fewer disability-free years.)

The report also included an analysis of comparative health status of adults (age 18 or older) based on self-rated health status, using the five-step, excellent-poor response options. They analyzed which factors were associated with respondents more likely to rate their health as fair or poor. The results are shown in figure 3.2.

Three groups are the most likely to report fair or poor health: blacks, Hispanics, and American Indians. These are the same three groups most likely to report not having finished high school. The report also looked at the level of fair or poor health based on level of education completed. As shown in figure 3.3, the results are as we might expect. As was the case in reporting disability, those with lower levels of education were more likely to report fair or poor health.

The report also looked at the association of disability status and having reported fair or poor health. Again, not surprisingly, there was a substantial difference. Of those reporting fair or poor health, 39.4 percent also reported a current disability, compared to 8.6 of those with health greater than fair or poor reporting a disability.

While women could expect an average of 2.9 years more than men free of activity limitations, there was not a substantial difference between men and women in self-rated health status: 15.4 percent of men and 16.8 percent of women reported fair or poor health. Zajacova and Hummer (2009) explored whether there might be gender differences in the association between race, educational attainment, and mortality rates. They analyzed these associations using a nationally representative sample of 700,000 white or black adults born in the United States between 1906 and 1965. Consistent with data above, they found blacks to have lower levels of education and higher rates of mortality than

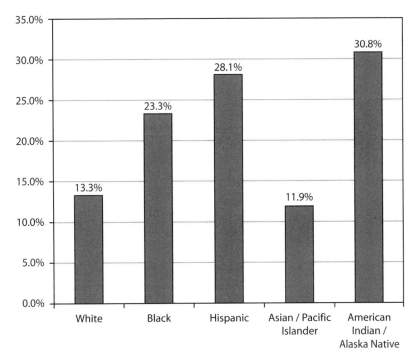

FIGURE 3.2. Percentage of Adults in the United States Reporting "Fair" or "Poor" Health, by Race/Ethnicity, 2010. CDCP Health Disparities and Inequalities Report 2013.

whites of a comparable age. However, they did not find major differences in the association between education and mortality rates for either white women as compared to white men, or black women as compared to black men. Blacks experience both lower levels of education and higher mortality rates than whites, but gender differences are not found in these associations.

Louie and Ward (2011) looked specifically at socioeconomic and racial inequality in the burden of disease and level of physical functioning in adults in the United States age 60 or greater. They found that those older adults with lower levels of education and lower levels of income were more likely to report impaired physical functioning. Without adjusting for education or income, blacks and Hispanics of Mexican ancestry were more likely than whites to report impaired functioning. After adjusting statistically for education and income, there

was no longer a difference in the level of impaired functioning among these racial/ethnic groups.

This finding for older adults—that race/ethnicity no longer had an independent effect on health status—is in contrast to the findings reported above that race/ethnicity continued to have an association with health status for adults age 18 or greater, even after controlling for education or income. Sautter et al. (2012) studied death rates of black and white men and women age 65 or older. They found essentially no racial difference in the association between education or income and the odds of dying among these men and women—with one notable exception. After the age of about 79, older black men with low income were *less likely* to die than lower-income white men. The authors suggested that by this age, more lower-income black men had already died, leaving "a relatively more robust

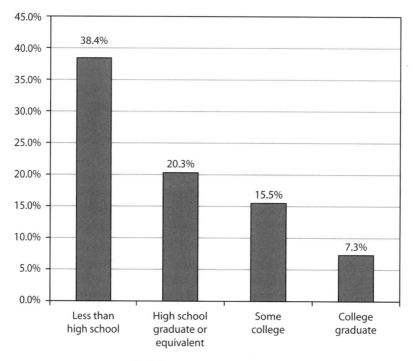

FIGURE 3.3. Percentage of Adults in the United States Reporting "Fair" or "Poor" Health, by Highest Level of Education Completed, 2010. CDCP Health Disparities and Inequalities Report 2013.

subgroup of black men and a black-white mortality crossover at advanced ages" (p. 1569).

Kimbro et al. (2008) confirmed the strong association between education and health for adults in the United States between the ages of 25 and 64, evaluating the associations for reporting fair or poor health, obesity, low levels of physical activity, and experiencing work limitations. They found strong associations between level of education and each of these outcomes. In addition, they found that blacks had higher levels of these adverse health outcomes than whites for all levels of education, while Hispanics differed little from whites at comparable levels of education.

The findings raise an interesting question. To what extent is the association between lower socioeconomic status and worse health outcomes in the United States different from that in other countries, based on each country's unique racial and ethnic history and current demographics? Martinson (2012) addressed this question in a comparison of the association between socioeconomic status and adult health status in the United States and England. Using nationally representative data for each country, she compared the association between income (measured in terciles) and a range of health indicators, including obesity, diabetes, high blood pressure, asthma, abnormal cholesterol, heart attack, and stroke. She found that "Overall, both countries had large, significant income gradients in health" (p. 2054) and that "Although the English enjoy better overall health than Americans, both countries still grapple with large health inequalities" (p. 2056).

As in the United States, the socioeconomic differences in health status identified in England largely reflect differences in health-related behaviors. As part of the ongoing Whitehall study of adults employed by the British civil service, Stringhini et al. (2010) looked at the association between socioeconomic position (measured based on occupational category within the civil service), behaviors, and death rates. They found consistently higher death rates among successively lower occupational categories. Differences in rates of smoking and patterns of diet and exercise accounted for approximately three-fourths of these differences in death rates. Looking specifically at older women in the United Kingdom, Watt et al. (2009) looked at the association between socioeconomic status (SES) over the life course and behaviors. They identified clear differences in patterns of diet and exercise among these women based on SES.

Substantial inequalities in health status based on income and race continue in the United States, but they are not unique to this country. While the level of education attainment explains much of these differences, in many cases black Americans experience more health inequality at a given level of education or income for many measures of well-being.

These inequalities are exacerbated by the lower level of educational attainment among blacks and other minorities. As shown in figure 3.4, blacks and Hispanics age 25 or older were substantially less likely than whites or Asians to have completed college or entered graduate school. Blacks and Hispanics were also substantially more likely to have earned a high school diploma but not gone on to college or never to have finished high school. Since educational attainment is the principal predictor of well-being as an adult, and blacks and Hispanics

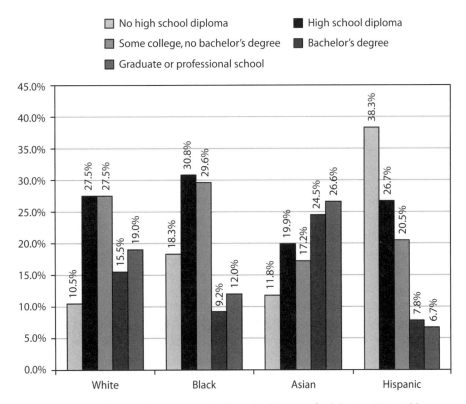

FIGURE 3.4. Educational Attainment in the United States of Adults Age 25 or Older, by Race/Ethnicity, 2010. US Census Bureau 2012.

TABLE 3.1. Children in the United States, Age 6–18, Whose Mother or Father Did Not Finish High School, by Race/Ethnicity (Percentages)

	White	Black	Asian	Hispanic	American Indian
Mother	4.6	12.9	14.6	39.3	19.4
Father	5.8	11.2	10.5	41.1	14.0

Source: National Center for Education Statistics 2010.

on average attain lower levels of education, we would expect these minority groups to experience lower levels of adult well-being, both economically and socially.

Lower levels of educational attainment as an adult have also been shown to have a strong association with the subsequent educational attainment of one's children. A report titled *Status and Trends in the Education of Racial and Ethnic Groups*, published in 2010 by the National Center for Education Statistics of the US Department of Education, reported that "Research has shown a link between parental education levels and child outcomes such as educational experience, attainment, and academic achievement" (p. 20). As shown in table 3.1, data from the report indicated that minority children were substantially more likely than white children to have either a mother or a father who never finished high school. This is especially true for Hispanic children.

Eccles and Davis-Kean (2005) reviewed the literature on the association between parents' levels of education and the educational attainment of their children. They found consistent evidence that the parents' education influenced children's education in multiple ways. One of the strongest was through the disadvantaged economic circumstances experienced by the families of adults with low levels of education. They experience both lower income and lower occupational position, both of which affect the circumstances in which the families live. Lower-income communities have weaker schools and other opportunities available to children. In ad-

dition, parents with low levels of education may influence children's educational aspirations through the attitudes they express about the value of education for their children. Davis-Kean (2005) found evidence of black/white racial differences regarding expectations about education verbalized to children and the frequency of reading to children.

These data add additional factors to the model described earlier in figure 2.5. While educational attainment as an adult is clearly associated with the health-related behaviors people adopt, and these behaviors in turn affect life expectancy, premature mortality, and level of disability, two factors are associated with some children attaining lower levels of education by the time they are adults: being of a minority race or ethnicity (in particular, being black) and growing up in a low-income environment. These two risk factors are associated, since minorities are more likely also to be living in the context of low income. These associations are shown in figure 3.5.

How does inequality in access to medical care affect health inequality?

Beyond the inequalities in education and income experienced by minority groups, there is also a long history in this country of racial and ethnic inequality in access to medical care. Since the early part of the 20th century the United States has elected to organize its health care as a market-based system. The principal means of payment for care is what has been re-

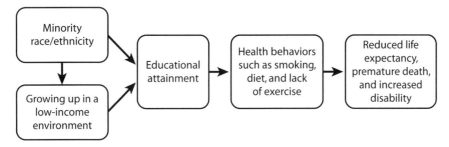

FIGURE 3.5. Economic and Racial/Ethnic Inequality as Precursors of Educational Attainment, Health Risk Behaviors, and Adult Health Outcomes

ferred to as "fee-for-service," in which health care providers charge a separate fee to patients for each service provided. Starting in the 1950s, many employers began providing health insurance to their workers as a fringe benefit. The federal government created a series of tax subsidies that encouraged the expansion of employer-based health insurance. For much of the 20th century the federal government played a relatively small role in the health care system.

In the 1960s the federal government took a major step to provide health care for seniors (age 65 or over) through the Medicare program and care for low-income families with children and those with disabilities through the federal/state Medicaid program. While these programs were largely successful, they nonetheless left substantial segments of the US population without health insurance, most of whom lack the economic means to pay for care through the fee-for-service system. By 2010, following the economic recession of 2007–08, 16.3 percent of the US population had no health insurance (US Census Bureau 2013b). The uninsured rate differed, however, by race/ethnicity. In 2012, 11.1 percent of whites and 14.6 percent of Asians were uninsured, as compared to 18.5 percent of blacks and 29.1 percent of Hispanics.

How much, though, does the greater lack of health insurance by blacks and Hispanics contribute to the racial and ethnic health disparities described above? Schroeder (2007) summarized the issue in a review article published in the

New England Journal of Medicine: "Health is influenced by factors in five domains—genetics, social circumstances, environmental exposures, behavioral patterns, and health care. When it comes to reducing early deaths, medical care has a relatively minor role" (p. 1221). Schroeder refers to a study by McGinnis et al. (2002) that described "A long-standing estimate by the Centers for Disease Control and Prevention [that] places the contribution of health care system deficiencies to total mortality at about 10 percent." McGinnis concludes that "even if the entire population had timely, error-free treatment, the number of early deaths would not be much reduced" (p. 83).

Of the remaining 90 percent of premature deaths in the United States on which improved medical care would have little impact, Schroeder describes behavioral patterns as responsible for 40 percent of total deaths, with disadvantaged social circumstances and associated environmental exposures responsible for an additional 20 percent of the total. Based on these data, it appears that despite the historical inequalities in the United States in health insurance and associated access to health care, inequalities in behavior and living environment contribute substantially more to premature death. These data are consistent with a study by Galea et al. (2011) that examined national mortality data for the year 2000. They concluded that of the 2.3 million deaths that occurred in the United States that year, more than one-third were directly attributable to forms of social and economic inequality, such as low education, poverty, weak social support, and residential racial segregation. Of particular importance in perpetuating racial disparities in mortality in this country is the continued pattern of residential racial segregation (Williams and Collins 2001).

The differing impact of low education and low income on the health of minority groups

The associations illustrated in figure 3.5 show the principal sources of disparities in health and well-being experienced by racial and ethnic minorities in the United States as well as those who grow up in disadvantaged economic circumstances. While these associations are accurate overall, some exceptions warrant further discussion and exploration. One of these exceptions is illustrated in figure 3.1 above. While the association between educational attainment and life expectancy is consistent for both genders in the three groups shown (white, black, and Hispanic), there is a clear hierarchical relation among these three groups. At all levels of education shown in the figure, blacks have lower life expectancy than whites, whereas Hispanics have greater life expectancy than whites. This is despite the markedly lower levels of educational attainment among Hispanics as compared to whites, as shown in figure 3.4. If low education is associated with reduced well-being in areas such as life expectancy, and Hispanics have substantially lower levels of education than either whites or blacks, then why is Hispanic life expectancy greater?

Infant mortality presents another area in which minority race/ethnicity has a differential impact. Low income and low maternal education are known risk factors for premature birth and associated risk of infant mortality. Hispanic women show lower levels of both factors than white women and lower levels of education than black women. However, in 2010, the infant mortality rate of infants born to Hispanic mothers was essentially identical to the rate for white mothers: 5.25 per 1,000 live births for Hispanics and 5.18 per 1,000 for whites. (Matthews and MacDorman 2013) By comparison, the infant mortality rate for infants born to black mothers that year was 11.46. For mothers giving birth as teenagers, one of the highest risk groups, the white infant mortality rate was 8.49, the black rate was 12.87, and the Hispanic rate was 6.22. Among teenage Hispanic mothers, those of Mexican ancestry had the lowest rate of all groups at 5.58 per 1,000, despite having some of the lowest levels of education and income of any group.

By contrast, obesity in the United States, one of the principal contributors to diabetes and its many complications, is more common among black and Hispanic adults than among white adults (Flegal et al. 2012). Among children between ages 2 and 19, 21.2 percent of Hispanic youths and 24.3 percent of black youths were obese, as compared to 14.0 percent of white youths (Ogden et al. 2012). Among children younger than 2, there was an even more striking disparity. Using a measure of high weight-for-recumbent-length, a common measure of excess weight among infants and toddlers, 14.8 percent of Hispanic infants were overweight, as compared to 8.4 percent of white infants and 8.7 percent of black infants. Mexican American infants had an even higher rate of 15.7 percent. For matters of excessive weight that places an individual at higher risk of multiple adverse health outcomes, blacks and especially Hispanics are at increased risk as compared to whites, consistent with their lower economic and educational status.

In addition to obesity and related issues of diet and exercise, smoking is one of the principal contributors to premature death and to increased rates of disability. As shown in figure 1.1, smoking prevalence is closely tied to educational attainment. Given that average educational attainment is lower among blacks and Hispanics in the United States than among whites, one might expect higher rates of smoking in these populations. This is not the case, however. In 2010, the prevalence of smoking among adults age 18 or older was 25.8 percent for whites, 25.4 percent for blacks, and 22.9 percent for Hispanics (Garrett et al. 2013). The highest adult smoking rates were among American Indians, with a rate of 34.4 percent. Among teenage smokers, American Indians and whites stood out with rates of 13.6 and 10.2 percent, compared to rates of 5.0 percent for blacks and 7.7 percent for Hispanics. Something more complex than simple racial or ethnic differences is affecting rates of smoking.

The association between race/ethnicity and well-being through the mediator of educational attainment is not a simple question of minority versus nonminority status. Some other aspect of race and ethnicity distinguishes different groups.

The origins and meanings of the concepts of race and ethnicity in the United States

The United States Census Bureau reported that in July 2012, the total population of the country was estimated to be 308,745,538. Of these, 50,477,594 were Hispanic, and 258,267,944 were not Hispanic. In a separate tabulation, the Census Bureau broke down the US population by race, as shown in table 3.2.

According to Census Bureau policies, people who identify as Hispanic may be of any race. Similarly, people of a given race can be either Hispanic or not Hispanic. As part of the 2010 national census, respondents were asked two questions about each member of their household:

Question 8: Is this person of Hispanic, Latino or Spanish origin?

Question 9: What is this person's race?

According to government policy, the issue of Hispanic origin is separate from the issue of race. While the category of Hispanic included several categories on the census form (Mexican, Mexican American, Chicano, Puerto Rican, Cuban, or another Hispanic, Latino, or Spanish origin), each respondent was tallied according to the ethnic dichotomy of Hispanic/Not Hispanic. Hispanic was not considered by the Census Bureau to be a race.

As for a person's race, the Census Bureau includes the five categories shown in table 3.2, plus a sixth category of "Two or More Races." In explaining these categories, the Census Bureau webpage states:

> The racial categories included in the census questionnaire generally reflect a social definition of race recognized in this country and not an attempt to define race biologically, anthropologically, or genetically . . . People may choose to report more than one race to indicate their racial mixture, such as "American Indian" and "White." People who identify their origin as Hispanic, Latino, or Spanish may be of any race.

In identifying the racial categories it uses in gathering census data, the website explains, "OMB requires five minimum categories: White, Black or African American, American Indian or Alaska Native, Asian, and Native Hawaiian or

TABLE 3.2. Annual Estimates of the Resident Population by Race for the United States, July 1, 2012

White	Black or African American	American Indian and Alaska Native	Asian	Native Hawaiian and Other Pacific Islander	Two or more races
241,937,061	40,250,635	3,739,506	15,159,516	674,625	6,984,195

Source: US Census Bureau.

Other Pacific Islander." *OMB* refers to the Office of Management and Budget, which is the federal agency charged with defining racial categories in the United States.

The categories listed above are based on the OMB policy set in 1997. In that year the OMB published a revision to the racial categories to be used by the Census Bureau and other federal agencies in gathering population data. The new regulations defined the following five racial categories:

- American Indian or Alaska Native. A person having origins in any of the original peoples of North and South America (including Central America), and who maintains tribal affiliation or community attachment.
- Asian. A person having origins in any of the original peoples of the Far East, Southeast Asia, or the Indian subcontinent
- Black or African American. A person having origins in any of the black racial groups of Africa.
- Native Hawaiian or Other Pacific Islander. A person having origins in any of the original peoples of Hawaii, Guam, Samoa, or other Pacific Islands.
- White. A person having origins in any of the original peoples of Europe, the Middle East, or North Africa.

These categories represented a change from previous policy. Prior to 1997, the categories of Asian and Pacific Islander were included in a single category.

The United States and its European forbears considered the different populations around the globe to be distinct subspecies of *Homo sapiens*. In a 1758 book titled Systema Naturae, Swedish naturalist Carl Linnaeus reported on his study of both plants and animals, seeking to establish a taxonomy of all animal life on the globe. In that book he identified what he believed to be the four subspecies of humans and provided what he saw as their defining behavioral characteristics.

- *Afer niger* (African black): impassive, lazy, crafty, slow, foolish
- *Americanus rubescus* (American red): ill-tempered, subjugated, obstinate
- *Asiaticus luridus* (Asian yellow): melancholy, greedy, severe, haughty
- *Europaeus albus* (European white): serious, strong, active, very smart, inventive

We should note that, with the exception of the Native Hawaiian/Pacific Islander category, the categories described by Linnaeus are identical to those used today by the United States government.

Johan Blumenbach, a contemporary of Linnaeus, differed somewhat in his human taxonomy, specifically in regard to how to categorize the peoples of the Pacific Islands, referred to by Blumenbach as the Malay (Marks 1995). Writing in 1781, he argued that the human species had five subcategories—the four identified by Linnaeus, plus the Malay. While Linnaeus identified these categories based on observed behavior, Blumenbach relied on differences in physical appearance without referring to behavioral characteristics. Thus, in making its change in policies regarding racial categorization, the OMB was shifting from the categories identified by Linnaeus to those identified by Blumenbach—both of whom were writing in the 18th century.

For much of the 20th century, many in the United States considered these racial categories to be separate biological categories, defined by distinct genetic differences. However, as human genome analysis became possible and scientists began to study genetic variations among different human populations, it became clear that there were no distinct and consistent genetic markers that separated these racial groups (Rosenberg et al. 2002; Rosenberg 2011). These genetic analyses demonstrated repeatedly that there is substantially more genetic variation among the individuals within a "race" than there is between or among "races." While it is often possible to identify the continent of origin of an individual's ancestors, that information provides little in the way of useful information about the characteristics that individual will possess based on his race. It is for these reasons that the federal government, as well as most scientists, recognize the racial categories used today in the United States as "reflect[ing] a social definition of race recognized in this country and not an attempt to define race biologically, anthropologically, or genetically," as described above. In contrast, in gathering its census data, the Canadian government explicitly excludes questions about race, instead asking individuals to identify their ancestry using a broad range of ethnic categories (Statistics Canada 2012).

The changing demographics of the population in the United States

While the categories with which we as a society describe and categorize people have changed relatively little in recent years, the makeup of the US population has been changing and will continue to undergo fundamental shifts. In 1980, the population of the United States was 83.1 percent white, 11.7 percent black, 6.4 percent Hispanic, 1.5 Asian, and 0.6 percent American Indian/Alaska Native. An additional 3.0 percent of the population was listed as "other races" (United States Census Bureau 1983).

By 2010 the population distribution had shifted to 63.9 percent white, 12.2 percent black, 16.4 percent Hispanic, 4.7 percent Asian, 0.7 percent American Indian/Alaska Native, and 0.2 percent Native Hawaiian/Other Pacific Islander (the new category created by the federal government in 1997 and formerly considered "Asian") (United States Census Bureau 2011). Over a period of 30 years, the Hispanic population had nearly tripled as a percentage of the overall population, becoming the second-largest population group in the United States. This pattern, of an increasing percentage of the population being Hispanic with a concomitant

decrease of the white and black percentages, is projected to continue for most of the 21st century, as shown in figure 3.6.

Between 2015 and 2060, the United States Census Bureau projects that the percentage of the population that is white will fall from about 62 percent to approximately 43 percent, while the Hispanic share of the population will rise from 18 percent to more than 30 percent (United States Census Bureau 2012). At some point between 2040 and 2045, the white population will fall to less than 50 percent of the national population, making the country a majority nonwhite country for the first time. This is, or course, considering the white population that is non-Hispanic white. A substantial share of the Hispanic population is categorized as white by race; however, in 2010 more than one-third of the Hispanic population nationally responded to the census question on race by indicating "some other race." Many if not most Hispanics consider their Hispanic ethnicity to be a separate category from those who are white. Thus again, it seems most appropriate to discuss the population on the basis of a single category of race/ethnicity, rather than dichotomizing these into separate categories.

Another aspect of the demographic changes expected to take place in the United States is the racial/ethnic makeup of children under the age of 18. In 2010 children made up 22.8 percent of the overall population. That share is expected to fall slightly, to 22.4 percent in 2030 and 21.5 percent in 2050 (US Census Bureau 2013a). However, the racial/ethnic composition of the children is expected to change substantially, as shown in figure 3.7.

In 2000, 17.2 percent of US children were Hispanic, while 61.2 percent were white. Over a period of 50 years those shares are expected to become approximately the same, at about 36 percent each of the child population. Following 2050, assuming no major changes in the projected rate of change, Hispanics will be the largest group of children in the United States.

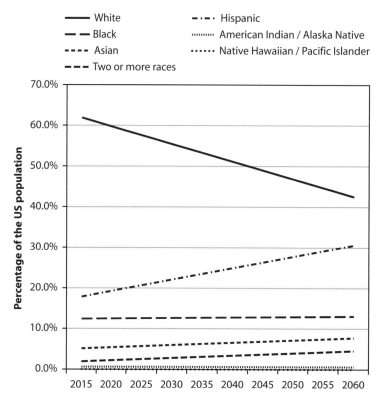

FIGURE 3.6. Projected Racial and Ethnic Distribution of the Population of the United States, 2015–2060. US Census Bureau.

As those children age, the graphs for overall population share of Hispanics and whites, shown in figure 3.6, is expected to intersect sometime after 2060.

The disparate impact of inequality on Hispanics and blacks

With the clear indications that the population of the United States will become, over time, increasingly Hispanic, how will that change affect the health of the population? We have seen consistent evidence that lower levels of educational attainment are associated with worse health outcomes. For example, the data in figure 3.3 above indicate a continuous, stepwise association between level of education and self-reported health status. Figure 3.2 above shows that Hispanics as a group report worse health status than all other groups, with the exception of Native Americans. Finally, figure 3.4 shows that Hispanics have some of the lowest educational attainment—especially at the level of not finishing high school. One might then conclude that an increasing proportion of the population that is Hispanic will likely lead to worse population health.

Using other measures of health status, however, calls this conclusion into question. As shown in figure 3.1, life expectancy clearly follows educational attainment for whites, blacks, and Hispanics. At all levels of education, however, Hispanics have a greater life expectancy than either whites or blacks, despite their lower levels of education.

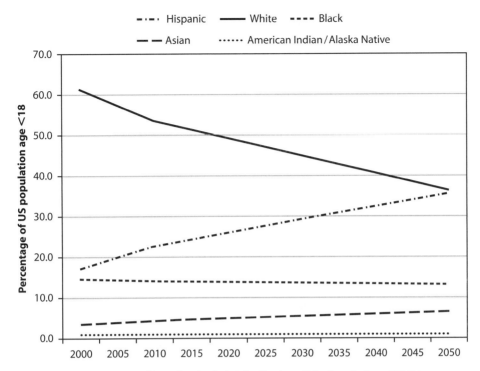

FIGURE 3.7. Projected Racial and Ethnic Distribution of the Population of Children Age <18 in the United States, 2000–2050. US Census Bureau.

Infant mortality is another measure that is closely associated with the level of education of the mother. Perhaps the greatest risk for infant death is being born at a low birth weight, defined as weighing less than 2,500 grams. In 2010, the infant mortality rate among infants born at low birth weights was 13.4 deaths per 1,000 live births, while the rate for infants born weighing more than 2,500 grams was 2.13 per 1,000 (Mathews and MacDorman 2013). Infants born at even lower birth weights of less than 1,500 grams had a mortality rate of 222 per 1,000. Nationally, 8.2 percent of all infants born in 2010 weighed less than 2,500 grams, while 1.5 percent weighed less than 1,500 grams.

One of the principal risk factors for having a low-birth-weight infant is low maternal education. In 2008 in the United States, the rate of low-birth-weight infants among mothers with only a high school diploma was 8.4 percent, of those with some college but no bachelor's degree 7.7 percent, and among those with bachelor's degree or higher 6.9 percent (CDCP 2012).

However, the association between maternal education and rate of low birth weight varies by the race/ethnicity of the mother. Looking at data for births to mothers age 20 or over (thus avoiding the higher rate of low birth weight among teen mothers), we see that Hispanics and Asians show a different pattern than other racial groups in the United States. These data are shown in figure 3.8.

Births to white mothers, black mothers, and Native American mothers show a consistent association with the mother's level of education, with lower educational levels being associated with higher rates of low-birth-weight infants for all levels of education shown. Births to Asian

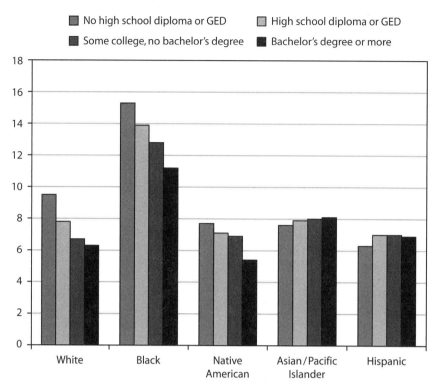

FIGURE 3.8. Low Birth Weight as Percentage of Live Births to Mothers Age 20 or Over, United States, 2008, by Race/Ethnicity and Educational Attainment. CDCP—Health, United States, 2011.

mothers and Hispanic mothers show no clear association between educational level and rate of low birth weight. In addition, despite having the lowest average level of educational attainment of all the groups shown, Hispanic mothers have the lowest rate of low birth weight of all the groups shown.

Another aspect of these associations warrants discussion. While it is the case that Hispanic mothers have the lowest rate of low-birth-weight infants despite their overall lower levels of education, these associations vary by the Hispanic subgroup the mother belongs to and the immigration status of the mother. In 2008, among Hispanic mothers, Mexicans consistently had the lowest rate of low birth weight, while Puerto Ricans had the highest. While the Mexican rate was the lowest of any racial/ethnic group, the Puerto Rican rate was consistently greater than either the white or the Native American rate.

Using comparable data from 1998, Acevedo-Garcia et al. (2005) compared these rates both by the mother's level of education and the mother's immigration status. They compared Hispanic mothers age 20 or older with other racial/ethnic groups, breaking each group down by whether the mother was born in the United States or abroad. For white, black, and Asian mothers, there was a consistent association between education and risk of low birth weight, with the rates for the foreign-born mothers somewhat lower than for the US-born mothers. For Hispanic mothers, however, the association between educational attainment varied by the mother's place of birth, with higher rates of low birth weight for lower-educated Hispanic mothers born in the United States but no educational gradient for Hispanic mothers born outside the country. Among Hispanic mothers, those with less than a high school education born outside the United States had the *lowest* rate of low birth weight of any group. There appears to be a powerful protective effect for foreign-born Hispanic mothers with low education regarding their risk of having a low-birth-weight infant and the corresponding risk of infant mortality. This association is often referred to as "the Hispanic paradox."

As described above, Acevedo-Garcia found a protective effect for black women who were born outside the United States but who gave birth in the United States (2005). These data are consistent with the data reported by David and Collins (1997) in their study of differential birth weights of infants born to black and white women in the period 1980–1995 in Illinois. Illinois had a long history of racial differences in birth weight distribution and associated infant mortality between black and white infants. David and Collins compared the birth weights of infants born to white mothers born in the United States and living in Illinois to those of two groups of black women living in Illinois: those born in the United States and those born in Africa. The birth weights of the infants born to US-born black women were consistently lower than those of the white women. The birth weights of the infants born to African-born black women were nearly identical those of the white women. The US-born black women showed consistent differences in behavioral risk factors for low birth weight when compared to the African-born black women, with a higher rate of teen pregnancy (28% US-born vs. 1.5% African-born), not having completed high school (36% US-born vs. 8% African-born), and being unmarried at the time of birth (76% US-born vs. 24% African-born).

Why do black women in the United States give birth to many more low- and very-low-birth-weight infants than white women? In a review of recent research on this question,

David and Collins summarized a series of studies that "showed an adverse impact of perceived racial discrimination on the birth outcome for Black women" (2007, p. 1195). Growing up in a society that has a centuries-long history of racial discrimination, principally against blacks, can lead to chronic elevation of the body's stress response and injury to the cardiovascular system, even at a young age. Thurston and Matthews (2009) studied the thickness and stiffness of the lining of the carotid artery of black and white teenagers with an average age of 18. They found that the black teenagers had increased levels of both measures, an indication of early injury to the lining of the arterial system thought to be the result of chronic stress due to a combination of low SES and racial bias targeted against blacks.

To what extent do young black women growing up in the United States experience a level of racial discrimination that black women growing up in Africa don't face? This was the question addressed by Dominguez et al. (2009). They surveyed 185 US-born and 114 foreign-born black pregnant women enrolled in an ongoing study of birth outcomes among women in Boston, Massachusetts. They asked subjects the extent to which they had experienced racial bias, either targeting themselves as an individual or blacks as a racial group. They found the odds that a US-born black woman had experienced individual or group racism in her childhood, respectively, were 4.1 times and 7.8 times those of a foreign-born woman. They found that African-born black women reported the lowest rates of racism during childhood, while Caribbean-born blacks had rates of childhood racism that were more similar to the US-born women.

These findings were for foreign-born woman who had emigrated to the United States after their 18th birthday. Foreign-born women who emigrated before age 18 were more similar to US-born women in their experiences of racism. These findings are consistent with the concept that the chronic stress of growing up in a climate of racial discrimination can harm the vascular system, with adverse consequences for vascular-rich organ systems such as the female reproductive tract.

Williams et al. (2007) looked at the differences between US-born and Caribbean-born blacks currently living in the United States in their prevalence of major depression during adulthood. While both groups had rates of depression that were lower than the rates among white adults in the United States, the Caribbean-born blacks reported significantly less depression than the US-born blacks.

Hudson et al. (2013) conducted a similar study, assessing the association between the socioeconomic position (SEP) experienced throughout the life course, experiences of racial discrimination, and two health outcomes: symptoms of depression and overall self-rated health status. They compared nationally representative samples of black and white adults in the United States. They found that those with lower SEP experienced depressive symptoms more often, as did those who experienced racial discrimination. In looking at the interaction between SEP and having experienced discrimination, they found that blacks with higher SEP reported greater levels of depressive symptoms in association with the experience of racial discrimination. Not surprisingly, higher levels of depression were associated with lower overall self-rated health for both whites and blacks.

If the experience of racial discrimination can affect cardiovascular health, birth outcomes, and mental health, how early does that experience begin to exert its effects on blacks in the United States? Sanders-Phillips et al. (2009) suggest that these factors begin to influence children early in the life course, with potentially harmful effects that may be lifelong. They suggest that

> A child's sense of control over life and health outcomes as well as perceptions of the world as fair, equal, and just are significantly influenced by his or her social experiences and environment. Unfortunately, the social environment for many children of color includes personal and family experiences of racial discrimination that foster perceptions of powerlessness, inequality, and injustice. In turn, these perceptions may influence child health outcomes and disparities by affecting biological functioning (e.g., cardiovascular and immune function) and the quality of the parent-child relationship and promoting psychological distress (e.g., self-efficacy, depression, anger) that can be associated with risk-taking and unhealthy behaviors. (p. S176)

They also describe the situation known as social anomie, "which is characterized by feelings of hopelessness and perceptions of little control over life outcomes . . . Racial discrimination increases anomie by reinforcing perceptions of inequality and limiting options for achieving life goals" (p. S178). These feelings of depression, anger, and hopelessness are associated with patterns of unhealthy behaviors, including higher levels of risk-taking.

Jackson et al. (2009) suggest that the unhealthy behaviors adopted at an early age by those facing the combined stress of socioeconomic disadvantage and racial discrimination act to buffer the physiologic effect of chronic stress. Such stress can lead to chronically increased allostatic load—the level of stressor hormones circulating in the body in response to environmental stressors perceived by the regulatory mechanism of the brain and autonomic nervous system. As described by Jackson and colleagues, "Although the stress response is well-adapted to deal with acute stressors, chronic activation of the system—as is often the case for those with poor living conditions and psychological stressors—results in poor psychological and physical health outcomes" (2009, p. 934). They suggest that behaviors such as smoking, overeating, drinking alcohol, and using drugs have a direct physiological effect of reducing the perceptions of stress created by a chronically elevated allostatic load.

Summary

The experience of inequality is directly associated with behaviors that impact well-being throughout the life course. The behavioral outcome with perhaps the strongest effect on well-being is the level of education one attains. For many outcomes such as infant mortality, life expectancy, and perceptions of well-being, those with lower levels of education fare worse than those from comparable backgrounds with higher levels of education. We find important exceptions to his association, however, when we also consider race and ethnicity. Many Hispanics in the United States experience better health outcomes than other groups, despite their relatively lower rates of educational attainment. This benefit is enjoyed principally by Hispanics who were born in other countries and then emigrated to the United States. As successive generations of immigrants experience and adapt to the dominant US culture, their patterns of dietary and other behaviors change, with consequent worsening of many health outcomes. The culture one grows up in has substantial impacts on patterns of behavior.

Perhaps one of the most harmful cultural effects is that of experiencing racial discrimination. Particularly for blacks born and raised in the United States, the racial discrimination that continues to pervade our society despite formal legal protections creates a combination of harmful physiologic responses and unhealthy behaviors that combine to affect one's physical and mental health throughout the life course, as well as the health of one's children.

In subsequent chapters we will explore the many ways in which humans learn patterns of behavior, both those that have beneficial effects on well-being and those that harm well-being. Some of these learned behaviors reflect psychological traits, and some reflect cognitive differences associated with early neurological development. Many of these early developmental processes, however, are directly affected by the cultural and social context in which a child grows up, the subject addressed in the following chapters.

REFERENCES

Acevedo-Garcia, D., Soobader, M. J., & Berkman, L. F. 2005. The differential effect of foreign-born status on low birth weight by race/ethnicity and education. Pediatrics 115(1): e20-30.

Centers for Disease Control and Prevention, US Department of Health and Human Services. 2012. Low birthweight live births among mothers 20 years of age and over, by detailed race, Hispanic origin, and education of mother: United States, selected reporting areas 2007 and 2008, available at www.cdc.gov/nchs/data/hus/2011/010.pdf, accessed 1/30/14.

———. 2013. Health disparities & inequalities report—United States, 2013, available at www.cdc.gov/minorityhealth/CHDIReport.html, accessed 1/15/13.

David, R. D., & Collins, J. W. 1997. Differing birthweight among infants of US-born Blacks, African-born Blacks, and US-born Whites. New England Journal of Medicine 337: 1209-14.

———. 2007. Disparities in infant mortality: What's genetics got to do with it? American Journal of Public Health 97(7): 1191-97.

Davis-Kean, P. E. 2005. The influence of parent education and family income on child achievement: The indirect role of parental expectations and the home environment. Journal of Family Psychology 19(2): 294-304.

Dominguez, T. P., Strong, E. F., Krieger, N., Gillman, M. W., & Rich-Edwards, J. W. 2009. Differences in the self-reported racism experiences of US-born and foreign-born Black pregnant women. Social Science and Medicine 69: 258-65.

Eccles, J. S., & Davis-Kean, P. E. 2005. Influences of parents' education on their children's educational attainments: The role of parent and child perceptions. London Review of Education 3(3): 191-204.

Flegal, K. M., Carroll, M. D., Kit, B. K., & Ogden, C. L. 2012. Prevalence of obesity and trends in the distribution of body mass index among US adults, 1999-2010. JAMA 307(5): 491-97.

Galea, S., Tracy, M., Hoggatt, K. J., Dimaggio, C., & Karpati, A. 2011. Estimated deaths attributable to social factors in the United States. American Journal of Public Health 101(8): 1456-65.

Garrett, B. E., Dube, S. R., Winder, C., & Caraballo, R. S. 2013. Cigarette smoking—United States, 2006-2008 and 2009-2010. Morbidity and Mortality Weekly Report Supplements 62(3): 81-84.

Hudson, D. L., Puterman, E., Bibbins-Domingo, K., Matthews, K. A., & Adler, N. E. 2013. Race, life course socioeconomic position, racial discrimination, depressive symptoms and self-rated health. Social Science and Medicine 97: 7-14.

Jackson, J. S., Knight, K. M., & Rafferty, J. A. 2009. Race and unhealthy behaviors: Chronic stress, the HPA axis, and physical and mental health disparities over the life course. American Journal of Public Health 100(5): 933-39.

Kimbro, R. T., Bzostek, S., Goldman, N., & Rodríguez, G. 2008. Race, ethnicity, and the education gradient in health. Health Affairs 27(2): 361-72.

Kochanek, K. D., Arias, E., & Anderson, R. N. 2013. How did cause of death contribute to racial differences in life expectancy in the United States in 2010? NCHS Data Brief, Number 125, July 2013, available at www.cdc.gov/nchs/data/databriefs/db125.htm, accessed 1/12/15.

Linnaeus, C. 1956. Systema Naturae. Photographic facsimile of the first volume of the tenth edition (1758). London: British Museum of Natural History.

Louie, G. H., & Ward, M. M. 2011. Socioeconomic and ethnic differences in disease burden and disparities in physical function in older adults. American Journal of Public Health 101(7): 1322-29.

Marks, J. 1995. Human Biodiversity: Genes, Race, and History. New York: Aldine de Gruyter.

Martinson, M. L. 2012. Income inequality in health at all ages: A comparison of the United States and England. American Journal of Public Health 102(11): 2049-56.

Mathews, T. J., & MacDorman, M. F. 2013. Infant mortality statistics from the 2010 period linked birth/infant death data set. National Vital Statistics Report 62(8), available at www.cdc.gov/nchs/data/nvsr/nvsr62/nvsr62_08.pdf, accessed 1/30/14.

McGinnis, J. M., Williams-Russo, P., & Knickman, J. R. 2002. The case for more active policy attention to health promotion. Health Affairs 21(2): 78-93.

National Center for Education Statistics, US Department of Education. 2010. Status and trends in the education of racial and ethnic groups, available at http://nces.ed.gov/pubs2010/2010015/, accessed 1/20/14.

Ogden, C. L., Carroll, M. D., Kit, B. K., & Flegal, K. M. 2012. Prevalence of obesity and trends in body mass index among US children and adolescents, 1999-2010. JAMA 307(5): 483-90.

Olshansky, S. J., Antonucci, T., & Berkman, L. 2012. Differences in life expectancy due to race and educational differences are widening, and many may not catch up. Health Affairs 31 (8): 1803-13.

Rosenberg, N. A. 2011. A population-genetic perspective on the similarities and differences among worldwide human populations. Human Biology 83(6): 659-84.

Rosenberg, N. A., Pritchard, J. K., Weber, J. L., et al. 2002. Genetic structure of human populations. Science 298: 2381-85.

Sanders-Phillips, K., Settles-Reaves, B., Walker, D., & Brownlow, J. 2009. Social inequality and racial discrimination: Risk factors for health disparities in children of color. Pediatrics 124(3): S176-86.

Sautter, J. M., Thomas, P. A., Dupre, M. E., & George, L. K. 2012. Socioeconomic status and the black-white mortality crossover. American Journal of Public Health 102(8): 1566-71.

Schroeder, S. A. 2007. We can do better: Improving the health of the American people. New England Journal of Medicine 357: 1221-28.

Statistics Canada. 2012. Classification of population group, available at www.statcan.gc.ca/concepts/definitions/ethnicity01-ethnicite01-eng.htm, accessed 1/24/14.

Stringhini, S., Sabia, S., Shipley, M., et al. 2010. Association of socioeconomic position with health behaviors and mortality. JAMA 303(12): 1159-66.

Thurston, R. C., & Matthews, K. A. 2009. Racial and socioeconomic disparities in arterial stiffness and intima media thickness among adolescents. Social Science and Medicine 68: 807-13.

United States Census Bureau. 1983. 1980 census of population: General population characteristics, available at www2.census.gov/prod2/decennial/documents/1980/1980censusofpopu8011u_bw.pdf, accessed 1/26/14.

———. 2011. Overview of race and Hispanic origin: 2010, available at www.census.gov/prod/cen2010/briefs/c2010br-02.pdf, accessed 1/26/14.

———. 2012. National population projections, available at www.census.gov/population/projections/data/national/2012.html, accessed 1/26/14.

———. 2013a. Children as a percentage of the population, available at http://childstats.gov/americaschildren/tables/pop2.asp, accessed 1/26/14; Percentage of US children ages 0-17 by race and Hispanic origin, available at http://childstats.gov/americaschildren/tables/pop3.asp, accessed 1/26/14.

———. 2013b. Income, poverty, and health insurance coverage in the United States: 2012, available at www.census.gov/prod/2013pubs/p60-245.pdf, accessed 1/20/14.

———. Annual estimates of the resident population by race for the United States, July 1, 2012, available at http://factfinder2.census.gov/faces/tableservices/jsf

/pages/productview.xhtml?src=bkmk, accessed 1/24/14.

———. What is race? Available at www.census.gov /population/race/, accessed 1/24/14.

United States Office of Management and Budget. 1997. Revisions to the standards for the classification of federal data on race and ethnicity, available at www .whitehouse.gov/omb/fedreg_1997standards, accessed 1/24/14.

Watt, H. C., Carson, C., Lawlor, D. A., Patel, R., & Ebrahim, S. 2009. Influence of life course socioeconomic position on older women's health behaviors: Findings from the British Women's Heart and Health Study. American Journal of Public Health 99(2): 320-27.

Williams, D. R., & Collins, C. 2001. Racial residential segregation: A fundamental cause of racial disparities in health. Public Health Reports 116: 404-16.

Williams, D. R., González, H. M., Neighbors, H., et al. 2007. Prevalence and distribution of major depressive disorder in African Americans, Caribbean blacks, and non-Hispanic whites: Results from the National Survey of American Life. Archives of General Psychiatry 64(3): 305-15.

Wong, M. D., Shapiro, M. F., Boscardin, W. J., & Ettner, S. L. 2002. Contribution of major diseases to disparities in mortality. New England Journal of Medicine 347: 1585-92.

Zajacova, A., & Hummer, R. A. 2009. Gender differences in education effects on all-cause mortality for white and black adults in the United States. Social Science and Medicine 69(4): 529-37.

CHAPTER 4

Society, Culture, and Behavior

The experience of inequality in the United States and its impacts on health-related behaviors reflect a number of cultural values. Concepts of race and ethnicity have come to be defined differently in the United States than in other developed countries, based on our unique history. As the growing number of immigrants in the United States leads to fundamental changes in our demographic structure, diverse cultural perceptions and expectations increasingly affect behavior. To further explore the link between behavior and well-being, we will examine the impact of cultural context on individuals, especially on children and young adults as they come to perceive their place in society.

The impact of culture: The Cultural Cycle

In their book titled *Clash!*, Markus and Conner (2013) suggest that, even though we as individuals often perceive our behavioral responses as consciously and intentionally driven, "psychologists have long known that most of what actually drives your behavior sails under the radar of your conscious awareness" (p. xviii). They instead suggest that our behavior is often driven by a series of nested interactions involving (a) our association with those in our immediate social environment, (b) our response to cultural institutions we have learned and internalized as part of the process of growing up, and (c) broad general ideas or concepts that create the structure for our culture and its institutions. Their model, which they refer to as the Cultural Cycle, is shown in figure 4.1. I explain each of the core elements of the model in more depth below.

The individual

The individual at the center of this Cultural Cycle includes the cognitive and emotional patterns a person has developed in combination with her or his personality traits and internal motivating

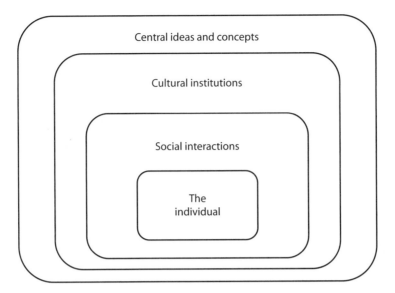

FIGURE 4.1. The Culture Cycle. Based on Markus and Conner 2013.

characteristics—qualities we will address in later chapters. Very often an individual perceives herself or himself as autonomous and independent of those around her or him. Markus and Conner underscore that this sense of an independent self is not universally held. The extent to which one perceives oneself as independent of or interdependent with one's social and cultural context differs across societies.

Social interactions

As described by Markus and Conner, our interactions are with others, "at home, school, work, worship, play, etc." (p. xx). Especially important for young children are interactions with others in the family. For the infant, this is principally the parent, often the mother. As we will find in chapter 9 when we discuss the development of cognitive abilities, the frequency with which a mother speaks directly to her young infant and the number of words spoken are principal determinants of the infant's language development. Similarly, the parents' response to the behavior of the infant—supportive for those behaviors of which the parents approve and

critical for those of which the parents don't approve—plays a major role in defining for the infant the optimal behavioral response to a certain situation. As the child gets older, siblings and other family members play an increasingly significant role in defining expected and appropriate behavior. (I can recall distinctly the behaviors my older brother defined as unacceptable for me and the actions he would take in response when I engaged in them.) As we grow older and spend more time with friends and age-mates in school and at play, we add other guidelines as to which behaviors are approved of and which are not. The behavioral expectations of our teachers play an important role here, although the teacher's expectations may be contrary to those of our friends, sometimes creating a behavioral dilemma. As we grow into adulthood these networks of social interaction grow to include those with whom we work and those groups with which we spend time (religious, sports, social, etc.). In each of these circumstances we become aware of the expectations of others as to what constitutes appropriate behavior in a given set of circumstances. Our continued membership in these social networks may depend to a certain extent on how well we follow these expectations.

Institutions

The concept of the cultural institution includes both certain organizational forms and certain rules of behavior. Those rules are sometimes written and formally adopted and sometimes simply understood, without the necessity of written instructions. As described by Markus and Conner, "Institutions spell out the rules for a society and include legal, government, economic, scientific, philosophical, and religious bodies" (p. xx). As described by Barr, "The concept of an 'institution' refers to the rules a society adopts that create its social, political, and economic structure . . . Institutions can be formal, as in written laws, codes of ethics, and prescribed procedures, or they can be informal, such as common courtesy and the strength of family ties" (2011, pp. 50-51). Nobel Prize-winning economist Douglass North referred to institutions as "a guide to human interaction, so that when we wish to greet friends on the street, drive an automobile, buy oranges, borrow money, form a business, bury our dead, or whatever, we know (or can learn easily) how to perform those tasks . . . Institutions may be created, as was the United States Constitution; or they may simply evolve over time, as does the common law" (1986, pp. 3-4). Thus, not only do we consider what types of behavior are expected by those in our immediate social context, we also take into account the formal and informal rules of our broader cultural group in choosing how to respond to a certain stimulus.

Ideas

The final layer in the Cultural Cycle proposed by Markus and Conner "is made up of the central, usually invisible ideas that inform our institutions, interactions, and, ultimately, our I's. Like the unseen forces that hold our planet together, these background ideas hold our cultures together" (p. xx). They suggest further that, while these central ideas around which cultures form are slow to change, they are subject to change. "You cannot directly alter the big ideas that animate the entire culture cycle, because they are so deeply rooted. But over time, as I's, interactions, and institutions shift, big ideas follow suit" (p. xxi). In the history of the United States and other Western countries, these "big ideas" that have organized our cultural cycle and that have changed over time in response to underlying changes in individual and group expectations include race and gender roles. Both were fundamental in much of American history, and both have altered fundamentally.

Differing perspectives on the nature of social structure

A number of sociologists have developed theoretical models of how these "central ideas" identified by Markus and Conner, as well as other core belief systems, have come together to create the overall structure of a society. While many of these models have aspects in common, others have fundamental inconsistencies. These classical theories of social organization include the following perspectives.

Conflict Theory

From a conflict perspective, the overarching structure of society develops as a consequence of struggles over power and influence. Many of the writings of Karl Marx emphasized competition among groups such as workers and capitalists over economic resources as central to the structure of society. A consequence of a conflict approach will be varying levels of social inequality due to the unequal distribution of resources within a society. A further consequence of this conflict over resources will be a lack of broadly shared social values. A common result of this lack of shared social norms is fragmentation of society along lines of class, race, and gender, with the inherent inequality these categories entail.

Functionalism

Nineteenth-century sociologist Emile Durkheim also wrote about the different segments of society, although he perceived them not as engaged in conflict but rather as parts of a stable, overarching social structure. A number of 20th-century sociologists have built on this concept, exploring the ways in which various components of society contribute to the overall stability of society. A key contributor to a stable social structure over time will be a set of shared public values and perceptions. Maintaining this ongoing social consensus will be a core responsibility of those in leadership positions.

Symbolic interaction

Originating with the writings of George Herbert Mead, this perspective on the origins of social structure suggests that people often rely on the symbolic meaning they perceive in the actions of others. People who observe behavior in others will often attribute symbolic meaning to that behavior, either positive or negative. As people come to interact with others, they incorporate into their actions both their intended symbolic meaning and their perception of the likely response of others to that action. How others respond to this action will determine the stability of the connection between these individuals, and ultimately between social groups. A common example given for the importance of the symbolic meaning of actions is the ways adolescents compare their own behavior to the way they perceive other members of their social group to perceive that behavior. If an adolescent perceives that his or her friends view smoking as a positive behavior, he or she may be more likely to begin smoking, even if he or she has learned the harmful health effects of smoking.

Each of these perspectives on the origins of social structure gives a central role to the institutions that are socially constructed by groups and societies. As described above, these institutions define the commonly understood rules for the creation of social structures such as governments or commercial enterprises as well as for the types of behavior perceived as socially acceptable.

The role of culture in influencing personality and behavior

In describing the cycle illustrated above, Markus and Conner define the concept of culture as, "the ideas, institutions, and interactions that tell a group of people how to think, feel, and act" (p. xix). We may perceive in the moment that our behavioral response in a given circumstance is under our individual control, while in fact our behavioral responses inevitably include cultural factors we have internalized.

The understanding of culture offered by Markus and Conner is similar to that proposed by Benet-Martinez and Oishi (2008). From their perspective, "Culture consists of shared meaning systems that provide the standards for perceiving, believing, evaluating, communicating, and acting among those who share a language, a historic period, and a geographic location. Culture . . . deals specifically with the values and norms that govern and organize a group of people (e.g., capitalistic culture), defining characteristics and behaviors that are deemed appropriate and inappropriate" (p. 542).

In most of American culture, when we are introduced to someone we have not met before and that person holds out his or her hand, we reciprocate by offering our hand to shake. We typically do this automatically, even though in doing so we are following cultural expectations. In non-Western cultures, it may instead be perceived as rude and perhaps offensive for a stranger to offer us their hand. There may be more appropriate, culturally defined ways to indicate to a

TABLE 4.1. The Key Differences between an Independent and
an Interdependent Concept of the Self

Feature	Independent self	Interdependent self
Definition	Separate from social context	Connected with social context
Tasks	Be unique Express self Realize internal attributes Promote own goals Be direct; "say what's on your mind"	Belong, fit in Occupy one's proper place Engage in appropriate action Promote others' goals Be indirect; "read others' minds"
Role of others	*Self-evaluation:* others important for social comparison, reflected appraisal	*Self-definition:* relationships with others in specific contexts define the self
Basis of self-esteem	Ability to express self, validate internal attributes	Ability to adjust, restrain self, maintain harmony with social context

Source: Based on Markus and Kitayama 1991.

stranger that we acknowledge and respect them. How enthusiastically or how hesitantly we offer the culturally appropriate greeting may reflect our individual personality in the context of that culture. Thus, "personality—the affective, motivational, and cognitive dispositions that influence our evaluations and reactions to the environment—cannot be separated from the broad social and cultural context in which it develops and is expressed" (Benet-Martinez and Oishi 2008, p. 544).

Culture creates specific norms of behavior, such as how to greet a stranger when introduced. Typically, culture also establishes certain central values that are shared by those within that culture. One key aspect of this type of culturally derived value is how to see one's self and one's needs in relation to others within the cultural group. Markus and Kitayama (1991) have explored the fundamentally different role the self plays in different cultural traditions. In their research they compared and contrasted the role of the self in the United States and Japan. They identified two fundamentally different cultural models of the relationship between the individual and the broader social or cultural group. They labeled these contrasting models as the "independent" view of the self (as reflected in US society) and the "interdependent" view of the self (as reflected in Japanese society).

Markus and Kitayama describe the concept of the independent self in the following manner: "In many Western cultures, there is faith in the inherent separateness of distinct persons. The normative imperative of this culture is to become independent from others and to discover and express one's unique attributes" (1991, p. 226). By contrast, the concept of the interdependent self, as reflected in many non-Western cultures, is based on the perception of "the fundamental *connectedness* of human beings to each other . . . Experiencing interdependence entails seeing oneself as part of an encompassing social relationship and recognizing that one's behavior is determined, contingent on, and, to a large extent organized by what the actor perceives to be the thoughts, feelings, and actions of *others* in the relationship" (1991, p. 227). The principal differentiating aspects of these contrasting models of the self are shown in table 4.1.

The independent person sees himself or herself as existing to a large extent separately from the broader social context. The tasks of an independent person are to be unique, to express yourself, to say what's on your mind, and to set and pursue your own goals, based on your own sense of self. You use the others around you as a basis of comparison and to get a sense of how you are doing. By contrast, the interdependent actor sees herself or himself as a part of, and not separate from, a broader cultural context. Her or his tasks are to gain a sense of belonging by trying to fit in, by speaking in largely indirect terms, and by acknowledging her or his proper place in the broader social structure. One acts as others expect and tries to place the needs of others ahead of one's own needs. The independent individual gains a sense of self-esteem by being able to express uniqueness, while the interdependent individual gains self-esteem by maintaining harmony in the relationship with others and by always remembering: "Don't make waves!"

Markus and Kitayama suggest that, across different societies and different cultures, "person is a social and collective construction made possible through an individual's participation in the practices and meanings of a given cultural context" (1998, p. 63). They also caution that, as scholars raised and working in a largely Western cultural tradition, we not simply accept the independent concept of self as the given norm. Nor should we approach the independent/interdependent contrast as strictly a contrast between Eastern and Western cultures. They underscore that, beyond being a cultural characteristic of cultures such as Japan, China, and Southeast Asia, interdependence is also characteristic of many areas of Africa and South America. Markus and Conner (2013) describe Mexican culture, both for those living in Mexico and for Mexican-Americans living in the United States, as heavily interdependent, with emphasis on characteristics such as *simpatía* (pleasant relationships with others) and the importance of *la familia* (the family). The importance of interdependence for Mexican-Americans presents potential problems for those living in the United States, where there often is a heavy cultural emphasis on independence. The issue of acculturation, or how one adapts to a situation in which both independent and interdependent

values exist simultaneously, has consequences both for behavior and for health outcomes. I discuss this issue in more depth later in this chapter.

The differences between those raised in an independent versus an interdependent context do not diminish the similarities in the process of growth and maturation children experience in different cultures. The early neurological and cognitive development of children born into different cultural environments are fundamentally similar. The role of hearing language as a basis for developing language, and the cognitive development of a sense of one's capabilities—as well as the vulnerability of this developmental process for children raised in neglectful or abusive circumstances—are largely the same regardless of cultural context.

While the underlying developmental processes may be similar in different cultures, the internalization of norms and values from the cultural context in which one grows up may still have powerful effects on how one responds to a range of personal circumstances. For example, Park et al. (2012) looked at how adults in Japan and the United States responded to stressful circumstances in their lives, based on their perceived level of social support from their spouse or partner, other family members, and friends. They evaluated the extent to which the stressful circumstances were associated with poor physical health (measured as the number of chronic conditions experienced recently) and self-rated health. For adults in Japan experiencing stressful conditions, perceiving stronger social support was associated with better health status than those reporting less sense of support. By contrast, US subjects demonstrated no association between social support and health status.

In another study comparing Japan and the United States, Kan et al. (2014) assessed how certain adult personality traits affected the well-established association between socioeconomic position (SEP) and health outcomes. SEP was measured in two ways: level of education completed and perceived subjective social status (SSS). They hypothesized that self-esteem, a characteristic more valued in independent cultures than in interdependent cultures, would show a stronger effect on the association of SEP and health status in the United States than in Japan. They confirmed this hypothesis, finding that "self-esteem significantly mediated almost all of the associations of education and SSS with self-rated health and chronic conditions among men and women in the USA, but very few such associations in Japan" (p. 53).

Miyamoto et al. (2013) took these analyses one step further, measuring the level of a physiological stress marker in adults in Japan and the United States who were experiencing negative emotions. Recall that, in many interdependent cultures, negative emotions such as sadness and anxiety are not perceived as demonstrating individual weakness. Rather, they reflect the need to adjust one's level of effort and to rely on the support of others. In an independent culture, by contrast, these types of emotions are often perceived as a sign of personal weakness or inadequacy. The body's stress response system is reflected in its allostatic load—a measure of the hormones and other bio-markers triggered by encountering stressful circumstances, either acutely or chronically. A chronically increased allostatic load has been found to be associated with elevation in certain markers of cellular inflammation in the body which, over time, can cause tissue injury. One of these inflammatory markers is interleukin-6 (IL-6). Miyamoto et al. measured the level of IL-6 in several hundred adults in Japan and in the United States. They also measured the level of negative emotions being experienced by these subjects, using a standardized psychological assessment tool. Among the US subjects, experiencing a higher level of negative emotions was significantly associated with a higher level of IL-6 in the blood. Among subjects in Japan, there was no association between negative emotions and IL-6. These findings were unchanged after statistically controlling for factors such as age, gender, education, lifestyle behaviors (e.g., smoking and obesity), and overall physical health status. Once again, psychological traits important to those in independent cultures, whether positive or negative, have a stronger association with health status than comparable traits in those living in a culture that values interdependence.

Other contexts in which independence and interdependence *Clash!*

As described above, Markus and Conner (2013) provided an extensive review of the range of social and cultural contexts in which independence and interdependence exist side by side, often creating potential conflict. These include the following contexts.

Gender

When my son was 2 years old, I had an experience that solidified for me the fundamental difference in gendered patterns of behavior, at least as manifested in the western United States. Whether due to the impact of the X:Y chromosome ratio or to parents' gender-specific response to infants beginning at birth, it seems that boy toddlers and girl toddlers often have a different outlook on life, and on the importance of connecting to other people.

While dropping my son off at his child-care center, I walked in with him to say hello to the teachers and to the other parents there. As soon as we got in the room, my son, clad in a diaper and a T-shirt, looked across the room and saw his friend Kevin playing with a toy truck. My son cried out a single word: "Truck!" Kevin looked back and responded in just as enthusiastic a voice, "Truck!" It only took a few seconds for the two boys to be happily pushing the truck back and forth.

Standing next to me, watching what had transpired between the boys, was little Emily, also two years old and also clad in a diaper and a T-shirt. When I looked down at her, she smiled, looked me in the eyes, and said, "Hi! How are you?"

How was it, I asked myself, that by age of 2, my son and his friend each wanted to see who could push the truck faster, while Emily wanted to know how I was doing? Markus and Conner offer an answer for my question. "If you thought that gender differences in selves and statuses arose mostly from biology, you could be forgiven . . . Rather than coursing through their veins, leaping across the synapses, or lighting up the cerebral lobes of men and women, the causes reside in the products and practices of men's and women's daily lives" (2013, pp. 48–49). It seems as parents, my wife and I had major roles in teaching our son to be male, to be strong and independent. Likewise, Emily's parents and the others who cared for her from the time she was born (e.g., child-care teachers) helped her to learn to look to relationships and to be sensitive to the needs of others. Again, as described by Markus and Conner, "Parents' different expectations for boys and girls emerge even before their children are born . . . When newborns greet the outside world, adults are standing by to shape the infants' selves in gendered ways" (p. 49).

It seems that, in the United States at least, girls are more likely to develop an interdependent perspective on their social environment, while boys are more likely to develop an independent perspective. These differences affect how boys and girls interact through the school experience, from their time in diapers through higher education. Once they attain positions of leadership, men and women have been shown to bring these perspectives to their interactions with others. When negotiating in a business environment, men often work for the "win"—the best outcome from their own perspective, regardless of how that outcome is viewed by the other parties to the negotiation. It has been shown, however, that while negotiating for a

"win" might lead to a greater outcome for the winning party in the short term, such a "win-lose" dichotomy leads to worse outcomes over the long term for both parties when they are required to negotiate repeatedly over time.

If, by contrast, a negotiator considers both his or her needs as well as the needs of the other party to the negotiations and seeks to optimize the combined outcome of both parties, these "win-win" negotiations have been shown to provide greater benefits to all involved. Perhaps not surprisingly, as more women have assumed positions of leadership and have brought a win-win, interdependent perspective to negotiations, both men and women have seen the greater outcomes produced by this approach, and many men have worked to learn and adopt this perspective on negotiation.

In her book *Secrets of Successful Negotiation for Women*, publishing executive Wendy Keller describes how "the people skills are the greatest asset in a negotiation, the ability to intuitively understand where someone is coming from . . . Luckily, they are the under-celebrated skills in which women tend to naturally excel . . . [W]hat woman wasn't 6 years old once and didn't realize that 'win-win' was the best way to play Barbies? . . . We already know it's about win-win" (2004, p. 17). She goes on to caution women that they may often have to work with "people who may not have our enlightened perspective" (i.e., men) but advises women to look for an outcome that gives these unenlightened others enough of what they want so they will come away from the negotiation feeling that they, too, have won.

Markus and Conner also emphasize the importance of the gendered differences over independence and interdependence for educational outcomes, especially in the areas of science, technology, engineering, and mathematics, often referred to collectively as STEM fields. They describe how, in both high school and college, "STEM is represented as an independent undertaking—the province of Lone Rangers and cutthroat geniuses who can abstract theories from applications and separate signals from noise" (p. 51).

Margolis and Fisher (2002) developed a study of computer science undergraduates at the Carnegie Mellon University (CMU) School of Computer Science. In the 1990s, officials at the school had noted that, of the students who enrolled in computer science as freshmen, fewer than 10 percent were women. Of those women who did enroll in computer science, fewer than half were still enrolled by the end of their sophomore year. The others had transferred to other parts of the University that didn't involve computers. By contrast, of the 90 percent of male entering students, more than 90 percent were still enrolled at the end of their sophomore year.

Between the years 1995 and 1999, Margolis and Fisher interviewed about 100 CMU computer science students, split evenly between men and women. In comparing responses by gender, they found that girls started relating to computers in fundamentally different ways than boys as early as first grade. Women described using computers as young girls for activities such as writing stories, while men described playing games on computers as young boys. By high school these differences had become more pronounced, with boys becoming more self-confident and more aggressive in using computers. Women described a male-dominated culture evident both in the high school computer science class and in the computer lab.

For those students who did enter CMU as computer science majors, study respondents described another cultural divide. As freshmen, men seemed most interested in learning the technical aspects of computer hardware and software, whereas women expressed a stronger interest in learning how to use computers to address social and economic problems. The introductory computer science classes focused heavily on the technical aspects of computing and had a strong male-dominant class culture, including the type of humor used in class by pro-

fessors. The women students described a growing sense of not belonging, with the result that most transferred out by the end of their sophomore year.

Based on these findings, the leadership at the CMU School of Computer Science made some basic changes to the way they taught students. They worked with faculty to increase awareness of the gender bias they had identified in the classroom culture and the differing perspectives of men and women students as to why they were studying computer science. They also focused on attracting women faculty and helping women students to form networks to be able to work together on instructional issues they encountered. After three to four years of these new techniques, they found that the persistence of women as computer science majors had risen to nearly 90 percent, comparable to that of men. In addition, as the word got out to high school students that women were feeling more welcome in computer science at CMU, the percentage of women in the entering class went from 7 percent to 42 percent.

Another STEM area in which women traditionally lag behind men in college is physics. Lorenzo et al. (2006) studied men and women freshmen students at Harvard University who had enrolled in an introductory physics class. They found that, coming out of high school, women students on average knew less physics than men students. By the end of the traditional lecture-based physics course, the gender gap had widened, indicating that men had increased their knowledge of physics by a greater amount than women as a result of having taken the course.

As a first step in addressing this gap, the physics faculty switched from a strictly lecture-based format to what they referred to as a peer instruction format, which interspersed short (10-15 minute) lectures with interactive, small group discussions of the issues raised in the lecture. After a few years' experience with this model, they went a step further, adding a weekly two-hour session in which students worked together in small groups, seated around tables, on a series of tutorials and hands-on experiments. This learning model showed a striking result. Despite women continuing to enter Harvard with a weaker knowledge of physics, by the end of the year-long physics class, students engaged in this "highly interactive" approach to learning no longer showed a gender gap in their knowledge of physics. Not only had the women students attained the same knowledge level as their male classmates, the men had also learned more physics with the interactive model than they had with the traditional, lecture-based model. The women, having started from a weaker place, had learned even more. From their study the authors concluded that "By creating a classroom environment that benefits both genders, the teaching approach described here improves student understanding and narrows the gender gap in physics education" (p. 121).

Data across a range of STEM fields have repeatedly demonstrated gender gaps in learning and a clear benefit to women students when the classroom incorporates interactive and supportive aspects. In a classroom environment that maintains its traditional independent culture, there is an added risk for many women students. By repeatedly experiencing lower learning outcomes and performance in STEM fields, many women may attribute these weaknesses to their own intellectual inadequacy. By resetting their own self-image at a lower level of intellectual capability, they may lower the goals and expectations they set for themselves, much in the same way that a reduced sense of self-efficacy can affect the goals one adopts (see chapter 7).

Social class

Anthropologist Adrie Kusserow has studied social class differences in the United States and suggests that there are class-based differences in perspectives on individualism that are every bit as important as the differences we discussed above between those in the United States and those in Asia and other parts of the world. From her study of children in New York City from different socioeconomic backgrounds, she cautions, "After many years of contrasting 'individualist' Americans with people from other, 'collectivist' cultures, social scientists are now recognizing that within the United States the meaning of individualism varies widely. We are also finding that not all communities practice, use, or socialize the same strands of individualism" (2005, p. 40).

Whereas children raised in the United States may still tend to be more individualistic than those in other cultures, Kusserow suggests that children in contrasting socioeconomic environments will likely adopt contrasting forms of individualism: "a 'soft,' upper-middle-class individualism, which focuses on the cultivation and expression of unique feelings, thoughts, ideas, and preferences; and a 'hard,' working-class individualism, which focuses on the cultivation of self-reliance, perseverance, determination, protectiveness, and toughness" (p. 40). Based on her study of children, parents, and teachers in a working-class area of Queens and in the Upper East Side of Manhattan, she contrasted these alternative manifestations of individualism, as shown in table 4.2.

Both children and parents from upper-class sections of New York City saw the world generally as a welcoming place in which children can work hard and expect success. Parents and other caregivers praise and encourage their children, careful not to lower the children's self-esteem through harsh criticism. By contrast, those in the working-class neighborhoods of New York saw the world as a potentially dangerous place in which children need to develop the requisite toughness to persevere through difficulty. Parents and caregivers use strong discipline to help the children develop resilience, given the uncertainty of what the future holds.

Children as well as adults who grow up and live in lower socioeconomic circumstances are well aware of the difference between themselves

TABLE 4.2. Comparing Soft and Hard Individualisms in Manhattan and Queens

	Soft	Hard
Individualism means	Emotional expression, creativity, uniqueness	Emotional control, self-reliance, toughness, perseverance
The self is	Delicate and full of promise, like a blooming flower	Hard and protective, like a fortress; strong and determined, like a rocket or Superman
Caregivers should	Give praise and encouragement, mirror emotions, foster creativity	Tease, discipline, toughen up, nurture without softening
Caregivers shouldn't	Damage self-esteem, block flowering of the self	Spoil or overindulge
The world is	Safe and welcoming, open to uniqueness	Potentially dangerous and forbidding, filled with ups and downs
The future holds	Success, personal achievement	Uncertainty, struggle, possible fulfillment (with hard work)

Source: Kusserow 2005.

and those in upper-class circumstances. They perceive not only economic differences but also overall status differences within society. Adler et al. (2000) showed a drawing of a ladder with 10 equally spaced steps to 157 non-Hispanic white women between the ages of 30 and 46 drawn from a range of educational and income levels. They asked the women to "Think of this ladder as representing where people stand in our society. At the top of the ladder are the people who are the best off, those who have the most money, most education, and best jobs. At the bottom are the people who are the worst off, those who have least money, least education, worst jobs or no job." They then asked each subject to place an "X" on the rung of the ladder that represented where she thought she stood in society. Most subjects placed themselves on rungs 5 to 8, with some as low as step 1 and a few at step 10.

The researchers then compared a measure of socioeconomic status that combined education and income to the rung marked by the subject and found them to be highly correlated ($r=.40$, $p<.01$). The authors demonstrated that, among these women, subjective social status, as reflected in the ladder rung they marked, "is strongly

linked to psychological factors that may predispose individuals to better health trajectories" (p. 590). Citing the work of Adler and others, Markus and Conner conclude that "People wind up viewing status, class, caste, and their consequences as natural and inevitable, rather than as human-made and changeable" (p. 103).

These differences in perspective based on socioeconomic position can have powerful impacts on students making the transition from a socioeconomically disadvantaged high school background to the highly competitive and individualistic environment of an American university. In an effort to increase the diversity of the student body, American colleges and universities often focus their admissions policy on disadvantaged socioeconomic background rather than an applicant's race. Many of these students selected for admission are of the first generation in their family to attend college (FirstGen). Many of these FirstGen students will experience a difficult transition into the college environment. As described by Stephens et al., "this adversity also stems from a cultural mismatch between the mostly middle-class, independent norms institutionalized in American universities and the relatively interdependent norms that first-generation students are socialized with in working-class contexts before college" (2012, p. 1389).

Stephens et al. conducted an experiment to test the idea that FirstGen freshmen students who perceived the university environment as clashing with their own perspective would experience a higher level of stress. They recruited about 80 incoming freshman students, roughly evenly divided between FirstGen students and students from academically advantaged families. All of the subjects were asked to read a welcome letter from the university president describing the experiences they would encounter as students. For half of the students in both groups, the letter described the university as a place where highly independent students will thrive. For the other half, it described the university environment as supportive of an interdependent, group-oriented approach to learning. Following this, students were instructed to give a five-minute speech to the group describing their own college goals. The researchers then measured the level of stress each student had experienced, using the level of cortisol in the student's saliva as an indicator of stress level. The students from the more advantaged background showed no difference in their stress level based on whether they had read the independent or the interdependent welcoming letter. By contrast, the FirstGen students who read the independent welcoming letter showed a significant increase in their cortisol level as compared to the FirstGen students who read the interdependent welcoming letter. As the authors described, "These results suggest that a culturally-mismatched environment—in this case, a mismatch between independent and interdependent cultural norms—can burden first-generation students with an additional, largely invisible layer of adversity . . . These independent cultural norms can be viewed as one important source of the middle-class cultural capital that helps students to navigate college environments"

(p. 1392). I discuss the issue of cultural capital in more depth in chapter 5.

Race and ethnicity

Race and ethnicity have always been powerful aspects of self-identity in the United States. In 1897, Senator Henry Cabot Lodge of Massachusetts stood on the floor of the US Senate and argued, "Surely it is not too much to sift now the hordes that pour out of every European steamship unsifted, uncounted, unchecked . . . The races that built up this country come in diminishing numbers. New races, utterly alien, come in ever increasing numbers." The "new races, utterly alien" the senator was referring to at that time were the Irish, Italians, and Jews. In 2014, the arguments heard on the floor of the US Senate were more likely to involve Mexicans, Hondurans, and Guatemalans, although the rhetorical descriptions sounded largely the same.

Race involves issues of physical appearance as well as ancestry from certain parts of the globe. In the 2010 census, the United States recognized five racial groups: White, Black or African American, Asian, American Indian or Alaskan Native American, and Native Hawaiian or Other Pacific Islander (US Census Bureau 2011). By contrast, Hispanic origin was considered an ethnicity, not a race. Within the category of Hispanic are multiple ethnic groups based on geography, language, and local culture, just as there are multiple ethnic groups within each of the groups categorized by the US government as races.

As reflected in the comments of Henry Cabot Lodge cited above, in the history of our country, the highest social status has often been given to those who are white—initially to those who were white and Protestant. As other white ethnic groups such as Irish, Italians, and Jews came to this country in increasing numbers, a new status hierarchy was created. Throughout this period, though, those of black African ancestry were consistently at the bottom of the status hierarchy—something blacks in the United States have historically been fully aware of. During later periods of immigration from Asia, Central Europe, and Central and South America, the racial/ethnic status hierarchy has become more complex.

As described by Plaut, the distinctions individuals make based on race and ethnicity, "are not simply natural, neutral, or abstract. Instead they are created and recreated in the process of everyday social interactions that are grounded in historically derived ideas and beliefs about difference and in a set of practices and institutions that reflect these ideas and beliefs and that therefore shape psychological experience and behavior" (2010, p. 77). Children growing up in the United States, regardless of their family's racial or ethnic background, learn these lessons, both consciously and unconsciously. Appiah (1990) has described the different forms racial and ethnic bias can take. He acknowledges that not all forms of bias are conscious and intended. Bias is often manifested unconsciously through the inappropriate application of stereotypes to individuals, or simply by a developing feeling of aversion or discomfort when encountering someone of a different race or ethnicity.

A person who grows up as a member of a nonwhite minority group will internalize a clear sense that he or she is different from whites. It is important for many of these individuals to maintain a sense of group identity with others of similar background. This sense of group racial identity encourages the development of a sense of interdependence that may coexist with the sense of independence learned from the broader US culture. When an individual experiences racial bias, whether consciously intended or not, he or she may experience the "Clash" Markus and Conner refer to when they suggest that "many American minorities have already developed robustly independent selves that travel alongside their interdependent selves. So their challenge will not be to cultivate more of

one self than the other, but to conjure more readily the self that best fits the situation" (p. 65).

The potential clash for minority students between independent and interdependent selves often occurs as students enter college, especially if they are transitioning from a socioeconomically disadvantaged background into a highly competitive university environment. As has been the case for gender, this clash often occurs for students of STEM subjects. Treisman (1992) described how, for many years at the University of California, Berkeley, a high percentage of black and Hispanic students who enrolled in his freshman calculus course would fail the course and as a result would be less likely to pursue a career that depended on a knowledge of mathematics. By contrast, the Chinese students who enrolled in calculus typically did well in the course. To see why the mathematical success of these two minority groups was so different, Treisman interviewed students from both groups.

For many black students, Treisman found the following pattern: "You wake up in the morning. You go to class. You take notes. You get your homework assignment. You go home. You do your homework religiously and hand in every assignment on time. You put in six or eight hours a week of studying for a calculus course, just what the teacher says, and what happens to you? You fail" (p. 366). Treisman noted that most black students approached this process independently. Rarely would a black student study for calculus with his classmates. By contrast, many Chinese students would gather together several evenings a week and study for calculus as a group, with each person contributing while also learning from the others. They would both learn from and support each other.

Based on what he observed in the Chinese students, Treisman began to work with black and Latino students entering his class, encouraging them to form study groups and to learn from each other as well as from the assignments. He also encouraged students to develop a sense of community based on a shared interest in mathematics. Treisman described the outcome:

> The results of the program were quite dramatic. Black and Latino participants, typically more than half of all students enrolled in calculus, substantially outperformed not only their minority peers, but their White and Asian classmates as well. Black students with Math SAT scores in the low-600s were performing comparably to White and Asian students whose Math SATs were in the mid-700s. Many of the students from these early workshops have gone on to become physicians, scientists, and engineers. (p. 369)

In much the same way that women at Harvard learned substantially more physics when the learning process was group-based and highly interactive, black and Latino students at Berkeley meaningfully improved their success in mathematics when they created an environment that fostered interdependent learning.

Acculturation: When people move across cultural boundaries

It thus appears that across gender, social class, and race/ethnicity, some individuals grow up and adopt an interdependent perspective on their role in the broader social and cultural context, whereas others grow up with an independent perspective. In a number of circumstances, including in particular the educational experience, these perspectives can clash, leaving some students feeling as though they belong in a position of advantage and others feeling a sense of disadvantage. How individuals perceive and respond to this potential clash of perspectives will affect the behavioral patterns they adopt.

Social scientists have been studying the issue of acculturation for decades. In 1936, a committee of scholars appointed by the Social Science Research Council offered a definition of the concept: "Acculturation comprehends those phenomena which result when groups of individuals having different cultures come into continuous first-hand contact, with subsequent changes in the original cultural patterns of either or both groups" (Redfield et al. 1936, p. 149). One can look at the immigration of Asians or Hispanics to the United States as a process of acculturation. One might also consider the entry of First-Gen students into highly competitive colleges and universities as a process of acculturation. In either case, how individuals and families respond to the cultural differences they encounter can have powerful effects on behavior as well as on well-being.

Sam and Berry (2010) have described different patterns of acculturation and their potential impacts. They identified four principal patterns of acculturation (p. 476):

- Assimilation: The "strategy used when individuals do not wish to maintain their cultural identity and seek close interaction with other cultures (or in some cases adopt the cultural values, norms, and traditions of the new society)."
- Separation: The strategy of "individuals who place a high value on holding on to their original culture and avoid interaction with members of the new society."
- Integration: -The strategy "used by individuals with an interest in maintaining one's original culture while having daily interactions with other groups—there is some degree of cultural integrity maintained, while at the same time they seek, as a member of an ethnocultural group, to participate as an integral part of the larger social network."
- Marginalization: The strategy "defined by little possibility or lack of interest in cultural maintenance (often for reasons of enforced cultural loss) and little interest in having relations with others (often for reasons of exclusion or discrimination)."

Based on the acculturation pattern an individual adopts, he or she will acquire different types of what Sam and Berry refer to as "sociocultural skills for living effectively in the new sociocultural milieu" (p. 478). The level of these skills one acquires will have a direct impact on one's overall sense of physical and psychological well-being and on overall life satisfaction.

Ahadi and Puente-Díaz (2011) studied how the acculturation process of Hispanic students attending a university in Texas might differ among individuals based on their differing personality traits, using what is commonly referred to as the "Big Five" personality inventory, described in chapter 7. They found that students higher in extraversion demonstrated a better adjustment to the cultural environment of the university, while those demonstrating higher levels of neuroticism experienced a more negative affect with more frequent symptoms of depression. The effects of these psychological traits appeared to be in addition to the effect of the type of acculturation experienced by the students.

Sam and Berry also underscore the potential role discrimination can play in the acculturation process, "with those experiencing high discrimination more likely to prefer separation, whereas those experiencing less discrimination prefer integration or assimilation . . . If immigrants experience rejection from the society of settlement, then they are more likely to reject them in return" (p. 479). As I discuss in the next chapter, the experience of discrimination can be a powerful influence on the behavioral response of an individual, especially a child or adolescent in the process of developing her or his identity and sense of self-efficacy.

The role of social networks in affecting behavior

From the above discussions we have learned how several factors combine to influence behavior. As described above by Markus and Con-ner, these factors exert their influence at the social, cultural, and institutional level. Thus the pattern of behavior one adopts as an adolescent or young adult, especially behaviors linked either directly or indirectly to well-being as an adult, will depend on a combination of the personality and motivation an individual brings to a situation as well as these external factors.

Mead et al. (2014) have described how various levels of normative influence coming from one's interaction with her or his social networks affect behavior, using as illustration the example of smoking behavior. They suggest that, especially with unhealthy behaviors such as smoking, social networks play a key role. These networks involve personal relations with others as well as more general social interaction either with individuals or with groups. From these networks, individuals come to understand the norms of behavior that are expected of them.

Mead et al. differentiate these social networks into two groups, which they refer to as *proximal*, involving principally family and close friends, and *distal*, involving neighbors, class mates, and others with whom one has regular contact without forming close personal bonds. The proximal networks tend to have more influence in setting behavior for younger children and preadolescents, as behaviors exhibited by parents and others one has come to trust play an important role in defining these behaviors as acceptable. For example, seeing a parent smoke on a regular basis suggests that it would also be acceptable for the child to smoke when he or she gets older.

Distal social networks often define groups and group membership that are separate and distinct from family. As one moves into adolescence and begins to develop an identity separate from family, it is common to model that identity on the social group or groups one either feels part of or hopes to become part of. For example, in the case of smoking, those who drop out of high school are far more likely to smoke than those who finish high school and go on to college. Independent of family, if an adolescent perceives herself or himself as similar to one of these alternative groups, she or he is likely to adopt the smoking behavior modeled on the perceived social norms of that group.

What if, though, the norms and expectations of the proximal network conflict with those of the distal network? If a teenager's parents try to discourage her or him from smoking while her or his peers are smoking on a regular basis, how does she or he respond? Mead et al. suggest that "When sources of normative information from the social network are in conflict, youth will often conform to the smoking norms and behaviors of their close peers" (p. 141). Of course, when both proximal and distal networks encourage smoking, the "risk of smoking behavior is maximized."

Beyond the influence of social networks, Mead et al. identify an important role for the broader environment in affecting behavior. The environment can be either physical or symbolic. In the case of smoking, the physical environment would include school, social venues, restaurants and bars that permit smoking, and places that sell cigarettes. The symbolic environment would include messages from the news media, tobacco marketing efforts, and sources of entertainment such as movies or television.

For many racial or ethnic minority groups, the symbolic environment would also include the presence of racial or ethnic bias and the extent to which an individual from a minority group has experienced that discrimination. Wiehe et al (2010) studied the association between smoking behavior and having experienced racial discrimination in a study of 2,640 low-income black or Latino adolescents living in large cities in the United States. For subjects between the ages of 12 and 15, there was no association between smoking behavior and having experienced discrimination within the previous six months. By contrast, black and Latino boys between the ages of 16 and 19 who had

experienced discrimination were significantly more likely also to report being current smokers. Interestingly, girls between the ages of 16 and 19 who had experienced discrimination were somewhat less likely to smoke than those girls who had not experienced discrimination. Gender plays a significant role in the ways in which social networks influence behavior.

In looking at the model described by Mead et al., we see a nested set of influences on individual behavior, beginning with proximal networks and extending through the broader environment. This model is similar in structure to the model of the Culture Cycle described by Markus and Cohen, illustrated in Figure 4.1 above. I have adapted that model in figure 4.2 to represent what I refer to as the Cycle of Behavior.

As individuals grow and develop, they turn to increasingly broad social networks for guidance in adopting patterns of behavior. As part of normal adolescent development, over time the distal network will often take precedence over the family and other aspects of the proximal network. Also, as one increasingly experiences the physical and symbolic environment, those factors also come to guide behavior.

While Mead et al. have examined smoking, this is not the only behavior pattern influenced in this manner. Dietary behavior and the associated problem of obesity are also influenced similarly. Beginning in early childhood, parents adopt their own expectations of what a healthy weight is for their infants. Often parents who themselves are overweight or obese have different expectations for their infant than normal-weight parents. (Hager et al. 2012) In addition, the culture in which the parent, especially the mother, was raised can have a powerful influence on perceptions of infant weight. Garcia (2004) described the disturbing interaction he had with a young Mexican American mother who brought her obese infant to the doctor because the mother was concerned that *no come nada*—"I can't get my baby to eat anything."

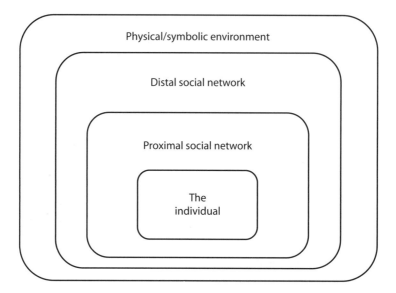

FIGURE 4.2. The Cycle of Behavior. Based on Mead et al. 2014.

National data has shown that, among adolescents age 12-19, obesity differs substantially by both gender and by race/ethnicity. In 2010 the highest rates of obesity were among Hispanic boys and black girls (National Center for Health Statistics 2012). The rate of adolescent obesity has also been shown repeatedly to be influenced by the physical as well as the symbolic environment in which families live. At highest risk are those who live in what are referred to as "food deserts"—environments in which food outlets such as fast food restaurants and convenience stores that carry unhealthy food and sugary beverages substantially outnumber grocery stores and other resources that are more likely to carry healthy foods such as fresh produce (Babey et al. 2011).

Summary

In the summary of chapter 2, we concluded that lifetime well-being is "clearly associated with certain behaviors, principal among them smoking, diet, exercise, and excessive alcohol use." These crucial behaviors are in turn influenced by the psychological and motivational characteristics of an individual as well as by the cultural environment in which that individual grows up and lives.

The cultural environment one experiences will carry with it certain rules and expectations about how individuals are expected to behave and what types of behavior are viewed as deviant. A central aspect of these norms is how an individual relates to his or her immediate social group, including family, peers, and members of a broader social network. Is the individual expected to see himself or herself as playing a role that is interdependent with the others in that network, or is he or she expected to establish an identity and a set of goals that is largely independent of family and friends? Different societies and different cultures offer different perspectives on these questions. A core aspect of these norms of social behavior is associated with socially constructed group identities such as gender, social class, and race/ethnicity.

With the pattern of social migration that is coming to be increasingly important in the United States as well as in other societies, a question arises: How does one interact with those from a different cultural background? Does one maintain his or her original identity, adopt the identity of the new cultural group, or find a way to do both? The answer to this question will be strongly influenced by the network of social connections with which one associates on a regular basis and by the social groups with which one comes to identity. I discuss the issue of group identity and its impact on behavior in the next chapter.

REFERENCES

Adler, N. E., Epel, E. S., Castellazzo, G., & Ickovics, J. R. 2000. Relationship of subjective and objective social status with psychological and physiological functioning. Health Psychology 19(6): 586-92.

Ahadi, S. A., & Puente-Díaz, R. 2011. Acculturation, personality, and psychological adjustment. Psychological Reports 109(3): 842-62.

Appiah, K. A. 1990. Racisms. In Goldberg, D. T., ed. Anatomy of Racism, 3-17. Minneapolis: University of Minnesota Press.

Babey, S. H., Wolstein, J., & Diamant, A. L. 2011. Food environments near home and school related to consumption of soda and fast food. UCLA Center for Health Policy Research, available at http://health policy.ucla.edu/Lists/Publications/DispForm.aspx?ID =8, accessed 7/22/14.

Barr, D. A. 2011. Introduction to US Health Policy: The Organization, Financing, and Delivery of Health Care in America. 3rd edition. Baltimore: Johns Hopkins University Press.

Benet-Martinez, V., & Oishi, S. 2008. Culture and personality. In John, O. P., Robins, R. W., & Pervin, L. A., eds. Handbook of Personality, Chapter 21, 542-67. New York: The Guilford Press.

Garcia, R. S. 2004. No come nada. Health Affairs 23(2): 215-19.

Hager, E. R., Candelaria, M., Latta, L. W., et al. 2012. Maternal perceptions of toddler body size: Accuracy and satisfaction differ by toddler weight status. Archives of Pediatric and Adolescent Medicine 166(5): 417-22.

Kan, C., Kawakami, N., Karasawa, M., et al. 2014. Psychological resources as mediators of the association between social class and health: Comparative findings from Japan and the USA. International Journal of Behavioral Medicine 21(1): 53-65.

Keller, W. 2004. Secrets of Successful Negotiating for Women. Edison, NJ: Castle Books.

Kusserow, A. 2005. The workings of class: How understanding a subtle difference between social classes can promote equality in the classroom—and beyond. Stanford Social Innovation Review, available at http://eahec.ecu.edu/smhp/smhpdocs/class.pdf, accessed 7/17/14.

Lodge, H. C. 1897. Senate speech, February 2. Congressional Record, 54th Congress, 2nd Session, vol. XXIX, part II, p. 1432.

Lorenzo, M., Crouch, C. H., & Mazur, E. 2006. Reducing the gender gap in the physics classroom. American Journal of Physics 74(2): 118-22.

Margolis, J., & Fisher, A. 2002. Unlocking the Clubhouse: Women in Computing. Cambridge, MA: The MIT Press

Markus, H. R, & Conner, A. 2013. Clash! 8 Cultural Conflicts That Make Us Who We Are. New York: Hudson Street Press.

Markus, H. R., & Kitayama, S. 1991. Culture and the self: Implications for cognition, emotion, and motivation. Psychological Review 98(2): 224-53.

———. 1998. The cultural psychology of personality. Journal of Cross-Cultural Psychology 29(1): 63-87.

Meade, E. L., Rimalc, R. N., Ferrenced, R., & Cohen, J. E. 2014. Understanding the sources of normative influence on behavior: The example of tobacco. Social Science & Medicine 115: 139-43.

Miyamoto, Y., Boylan, J. M., Coe, C. L., et al. 2013. Negative emotions predict elevated interleukin-6 in the United States but not in Japan. Brain, Behavior, and Immunity 34: 79-85.

National Center for Health Statistics. 2012. Prevalence of obesity among persons aged 12-19 years, by race/ethnicity and sex—National Health and Nutrition Examination Survey, United States, 2009-2010. Morbidity and Mortality Weekly Report 61(9): 165.

North, D. C. 1986. Institutions, Institutional Change and Economic Performance. New York: Cambridge University Press.

Park, J., Kitayama, S., Karasawa, M., et al. 2012. Clarifying the links between social support and health: Culture, stress, and neuroticism matter. Journal of Health Psychology 18(2): 226-35.

Plaut, V. C. 2010. Diversity science: Why and how difference makes a difference. Psychological Inquiry 21(2): 77-99.

Redfield, R., Linton, R., & Herskovits, M. J. 1936. Memorandum for the study of acculturation. American Anthropologist 38(1): 149-52.

Sam, D. L., & Berry, J. W. 2010. Acculturation: When individuals and groups of different cultural backgrounds meet. Perspectives on Psychological Science 5(4): 472-81.

Stephens, N. C., Townsend, S. S. M., Markus, H. R., & Phillips, L. T. 2012. A cultural mismatch: Independent cultural norms produce greater increases in cortisol and more negative emotions among first-generation college students. Journal of Experimental Social Psychology 48(6): 1389-93.

Treisman, U. 1992. Studying students studying calculus: A look at the lives of minority mathematics students in college. The College Mathematics Journal 23(5): 362-72.

US Census Bureau. 2011. 2010 census briefs—Overview of race and Hispanic origin: 2010. Available at www.census.gov/prod/cen2010/briefs/c2010br-02.pdf, accessed 7/17/14.

Wiehe, S. E., Aalsma, M. C., Liu, G. C., & Fortenberry, J. D. 2010. Gender differences in the association between perceived discrimination and adolescent smoking. American Journal of Public Health 100(3): 510-16.

CHAPTER 5

Identity and Behavior

Developmental experiences during childhood and adolescence have a range of effects on how the individual preparing to enter adulthood comes to view himself or herself as well as the world more broadly. As discussed in chapter 4, the cultural context in which one grows up can have powerful influences on these perceptions. The social environment in which one lives and works is also a major aspect of that world. As a central part of that environment, the social groups with which one interacts play an important role.

Social identity: Responding to the social group

When one moves from adolescence into adulthood, whether through a process that involves education beyond high school or through employment and similar activities oriented toward providing for one's needs, one will interact with others on an increasing basis. The social groups with which one interacts may be formal, such as other employees within a work group or other members of a religious or civic group, or they may be informal, such as neighbors and other acquaintances. To a certain extent, which will vary from person to person, individuals may come to define themselves based on the social groups with which they interact on a regular basis.

Individuals develop their identity based on how they perceive themselves independently from any group, in combination with how they perceive themselves as a member of defined social groups. To a large extent, it is this membership in groups that defines their place in society. To feel as though one is a member of a group, it may be necessary to adopt certain goals shared by the group. Accordingly, one will integrate the individual values and motivations developed as a youth with those held by the group. Tajfel and Turner have described this process as one of establishing a "social identity", which "consists of those aspects of an individual's self-image that derive from the social categories to which he perceives himself as belonging" (1986, p. 16). As discussed below, it is a natural tendency of social groups to compare themselves to other groups that have adopted different attributes and characteristics of group membership, and to create boundaries between theirs as the "in-group" and other groups as "out-groups." Being a member of an in-group caries more status than that enjoyed by those in the out-group. Groups then rank themselves and their members based on this perceived status. This competition for status can easily lead to intergroup conflict.

Walton and Cohen have described how one comes to share values and motivations with a social group. They underscore the influence of this social identity and suggest, "that people develop interests with and from others to whom they are socially connected" (2011b, p. 84). Individuals who see themselves as group members and draw value from that membership will be more likely to adopt behaviors shared by others in the group, whether beneficial or harmful to well-being.

Walton and Cohen acknowledge that this powerful influence of group membership on individual behavior is contrary to Western norms of independence. They suggest that "People from Western cultures perform a balancing act. On the one hand they have a great need to belong . . . On the other hand, they maintain an 'independent' self-concept, seeing themselves as agentic and unique" (2011b, p. 94). These forces of independent actions versus following group norms can potentially come into conflict when someone joins a social group but is unsure whether he or she has been fully accepted as a member. This can often happen when one is of a different race, ethnicity, or socioeconomic background from that which predominates within the group. Walton and Cohen describe how this issue often comes up in the context of higher education, a subject I discuss later in this chapter.

Alternative forms of capital and their impacts on social status

The concept of capital has been studied by social scientists for more than a century. When most people think of capital, they think of economic capital, the economic resources one possesses that can, when needed, be converted to money. Sociologist Pierre Bourdieu (1986) suggested that capital can exist in multiple ways. All the various forms of capital can be accumulated through labor, can be used to influence others, and can be passed to descendants. He wrote that "the structure of the distribution of the different types and subtypes of capital at a given moment in time represents the immanent structure of the social world" (p. 242).

In addition to economic capital, Bourdieu posited that individuals also possess cultural capital, often in the form of educational qualifications that can be used for economic gain, and social capital, based on social connections and the social status those connections imbue. He suggests that the different types of capital—"or power, which amounts to the same thing" (p. 243)—can often be used interchangeably. Bourdieu described cultural capital as existing in three different states: the embodied state, reflected in one's acquired knowledge or talents; the objectified state, reflected in one's material objects such as books or works of art; and the institutionalized state, typically reflected in certificates of academic or professional qualifications, such as academic degrees or professional licenses.

Social capital, on the other hand, derives largely from the social connections and contacts one has. As described by Bourdieu, "Social capital is the aggregate of the actual or potential resources which are linked to possession of a durable network of more or less institutionalized relationships of mutual acquaintance and recognition—or, in other words, to membership in a group" (p. 248). The more social network connections one has, and the more one can draw on those connections to gain needed resources, the more social capital one possesses.

Two aspects of these forms of capital are of particular interest from the perspective of understanding behavior. First, there is a certain degree of interchangeability among them. Those with greater economic capital can acquire greater cultural capital through the expenditure of the economic resources. Similarly, those with greater cultural capital, at least as perceived by others, may find it easier to create and then draw upon social network connections. The second aspect is that these forms of capital are often transmissible across generations. Economic capital can simply be passed on to one's heirs as a formal inheritance. As we have seen, cultural capital in its various forms can be transmitted to the next generation through supporting the development in one's children of a sense of self-efficacy and belief in the value of education, a significant part of which is the availability and regular use of books. Similarly, children often have as friends the children of those who are socially connected to their parents.

The greater one's capital in its various forms, the greater will, in all likelihood, be one's status within the community. Just as the possession of social and cultural capital can provide status, their relative absence can result in stigma. As described originally by Berger et al. (1977) certain characteristics of individuals, largely as perceived by others, will create a hierarchy of status within a community or a society. Examples of these status characteristics include race, gender, and the various forms of capital described by Bourdieu.

Phelan et al. have suggested that an individual's combination of status characteristics essentially creates that individual's rank in a community or society "based on the esteem in which the person is held by self and others . . . Members of a group form expectations about each other's competence to contribute to group goals based on their status characteristics" (2014, p. 16). Based on these perceptions, an individual

of low perceived status is also expected to be less competent and to act in ways that either do not support or actually challenge goals held by the larger group. Accordingly these individuals are often perceived in a position of stigma rather than status. As status characteristics are perceived both by others and by the individual possessing them, a negative sense of self will often be internalized by the individual who has been stigmatized by others. This stigmatized position can result in reduced well-being through a combination of experiencing increased stress over time and increased likelihood of adopting unhealthy behaviors in response.

Questioning one's identity in the context of cultural mismatch: The case of FirstGen students entering college

As described in the previous chapter, colleges and universities have been shifting the focus of their efforts to enhance the diversity of their students. For a period of time following the 1960s, diversity was seen largely as an issue of race and ethnicity and was addressed by affirmative action programs. Largely as a result of a series of US Supreme Court decisions, colleges and universities have been moving away from race as a principal marker of diversity, looking instead at students' socioeconomic status. As part of this effort, many academic institutions have been focusing on attracting talented students who are the first generation in their family to attend college. Often referred to as FirstGen students, many of these students are members of racial and ethnic minority groups, many come from relatively weaker public high schools in lower-income communities, and many are from immigrant families.

Individuals transitioning into adulthood look to their social and cultural environment for messages that both inform their sense of identity and provide guidance as to expected behavior. The transition into college, especially into a highly competitive college or university, can present substantial challenges for many First-Gen students. As Markus and Conner described (2013; see chapter 4), those from immigrant and lower-income families often grow up having internalized the cultural message that they are part of a group, such as family or community, and need to act in ways that best support the group. If colleges in their welcoming messages and professors in their classroom instruction suggest that students need to be independent thinkers, it often raises the question for First-Gen students, "Do I belong here?"

Another challenge these students often confront is a perceived gap in social and cultural capital when they compare themselves to other students entering with them. "Prior to college, [FirstGen students] have less exposure and access to the types of middle-class cultural capital—understandings of the rules of the game—that are taken for granted as normative by many American universities. Consequently, first-generation students are often uncertain about the 'right' way to act as college students and begin to question whether they belong and can be successful in college settings" (Stephens et al. 2012, p. 1180).

This mismatch in experiences and in social and cultural capital may also make it difficult for FirstGen and other students from disadvantaged backgrounds to form new social networks with other students at college. Without these networks, students may feel more isolated in the classroom environment as well as in the range of extracurricular activities available to students. Unfortunately, the result of this lack of connection and feeling of cultural isolation is associated with lower academic performance among FirstGen students. Stephens et al. describe a three-step process by which this "cultural mismatch" exerts its effects: first, the FirstGen or otherwise disadvantaged students initially feels out of place and uncomfortable in the university environment; as a result of this discomfort and the lack of social connection that goes with it, the student finds the assigned

tasks more difficult; finally, the student tends to perform less well academically than he or she is otherwise capable of. This weak academic performance can then reinforce the sense of cultural mismatch and isolation, often leading to continued academic difficulty and an increased risk of leaving the college or university.

Stephens et al. demonstrated that when FirstGen students were introduced to the university environment as one that supported an interdependent approach to education and explicitly encouraged to view the university as a "learning community," to connect to their fellow students as well as faculty, and to form learning groups with other students to support each other in assigned work, they found tasks assigned to them to be less difficult and showed improved performance as compared to First-Gen students who had not received comparable support and encouragement.

In a separate study, Stephens et al. (2014) identified FirstGen students entering a private university, most of whom were from low-income families, and during the orientation period to the university invited them to attend a panel discussion with a socially diverse group of senior students to introduce them to the college environment. Half of the students heard from the student panelists that they had used their cultural and social background to find stronger connections with others at the university and to improve their academic skills. The other half heard a similar panel describe how individual actions or behaviors had helped them succeed, without reference to the importance of forming group connections. By the end of their freshman year, the FirstGen students who heard the panel that encouraged social connection and group academic work had higher grades than the students hearing the panel that emphasized individual action, and they also had shown a greater tendency to seek out help from other students or faculty throughout the year. From these results the authors concluded that "The intervention provided students with the critical insight that people's different backgrounds matter and that people with backgrounds like theirs can succeed when they use the right kinds of tools and strategies" (p. 949).

In a similar study, Walton and Cohen (2011a) focused on African American students entering a selective college. Independently of FirstGen background, many black students experience a similar form of cultural mismatch, stigmatization, and social exclusion when they enter college, based largely on their racial differences with the majority of other students at the college. Due largely to what has come to be referred to as stereotype threat (discussed below), these students often do less well academically than comparably talented students who are not black. The researchers had half of the students read a report from the university that indicated that all students, independent of race, experience potential difficulty in the transition to college and yet are able to overcome it through a combination of individual effort and social support. The other half of the students read a comparable report that talked about other aspects of the college transition but left out reference to the commonality of overcoming initial personal and academic difficulties. They also had a group of entering white students read the same reports. They followed the students for a period of three years during college, comparing their grade point average, their self-reports of feeling a sense of belonging, their sense of self-doubt, their experience of feeling negatively stereotyped, and their overall physical and emotional health status. The black students who had read the report on the commonality yet transience of initial personal difficulties in college did better on all of these measures than the black students who read the other report. By contrast, there was no difference on these outcomes between the white students who had read the report describing common difficulties and the white students who had read the other report. Combined with the studies described above, these results confirm that students entering college from a disadvantaged socioeconomic or racial background are vulnerable to feelings of cultural exclusion, self-doubt, and resultant academic difficulties that can be averted through well-designed messages of inclusion.

The competition for status: Group identity, bias, and stereotype threat

As discussed above, in describing the creation of social identity, Tajfel and Turner (1986) underscored the importance of group membership and the process by which different social groups compete for status, with individual group members benefiting in their own identity based on the status that comes with group membership. This competitive process can easily lead to antagonism between groups perceived as dominant and subordinate. Individuals within one group can easily develop prejudice against members of a competing group seen as subordinate, with the consequence that "the more intense is an intergroup conflict, the more likely it is that the individuals who are members of the opposite groups will behave toward each other as a function of their respective group memberships, rather than in terms of their individual characteristics or interindividual relationships" (p. 8).

Berger et al. developed a theory of "status characteristics" by which "differences in cognitions and evaluations of individuals, or social types of them, become the basis of differences in the stable and observable features of social interaction" (1977, p. 3). They identify three basic characteristics used to define relative status under this theory: sex (today more commonly referred to as gender), race, and socioeconomic status (operationalized under their theory as occupational status). They point out that most of the characteristics attributed to different groups are "socially constructed," in that they exist based on social convention rather than biological differences and as such are adopted as part of the learning and socialization process of childhood and adolescent development. Based on characteristics attributed to specific groups (women as compared to men, blacks as compared to whites, lower-class individuals as compared to upper-class ones), people come to expect individual members of a group to exhibit the traits attributed to the group overall. A common example is the traditional expectation (since proven wrong) that girls and women, based on their gender, are not as capable in mathematics as are boys and men. Based on this expectation, school teachers would often approach a girl in their class as less capable in math than the boys. The girl was at risk of internalizing this clear message from her teacher and devaluing her own ability in math. This internal devaluation would often result in lower performance in math, thus confirming the teacher's stereotype of girls as less capable. As described below, this process of consciously or unconsciously internalizing a negative stereotype about intellectual abilities has been shown to exist in a range of groups and has been come to be referred to as both stereotype threat and identity threat.

In the United States, race has historically been a status characteristic that has both defined group superiority/inferiority and been applied stereotypically to members of a group, attributing to them as individuals the characteristics associated with the group. For those of us who grew up in the 1960s in the United States, the growing availability of nationally televised news introduced us graphically to the forms this racial bias can take. I can remember sitting next to my grandfather (he lived next door and had the only TV in the family) on May 23, 1963, and watching television coverage of the response of the white authorities in Birmingham, Alabama, to the black children who were marching in support of Martin Luther King Jr., who had been imprisoned because of his own participation in civil rights demonstrations. The police chief in Birmingham was a high school dropout named Theophilus Eugene "Bull" Connor. When a group of more than a thousand children, ranging in age from 6 to 18 years, began their march

from a park in Birmingham toward the downtown area, Connor instructed the firefighters under his command to turn their high-powered fire hoses on the child demonstrators and for the police to use their attack dogs. Images of these children being hit with the blast of the fire hoses and being attacked by police dogs were carried on nationwide TV, including the TV in our living room. The horror many in the nation felt at seeing the response of the racist white power system to these children was a major factor in the subsequent approval in Congress of the Civil Rights Act of 1964, the first major civil rights legislation approved by the US Congress.

Since the 1960s, a range of civil rights laws has been passed to protect the rights of blacks and other previously marginalized groups. While the type of racist behavior exhibited in 1963 by Bull Conner has largely disappeared, those who study racial bias have described other forms in which prejudicial beliefs have been applied to the detriment of blacks and other minorities. Appiah differentiated "extrinsic racism," such as that enacted by Bull Connor, from other forms of racial prejudice. He stated that "extrinsic racists make moral distinctions between members of different races because they believe that racial essence entails certain morally relevant qualities. The basis for the extrinsic racist's discrimination between people is their belief that members of different races differ in respects that *warrant* the differential treatment" (1990, p. 5). By contrast, those who exhibit what Appiah referred to as "intrinsic" racial bias do not consciously apply moral judgment to blacks or other racial groups. Nonetheless, they continue to apply negative expectations to individual members of that group, albeit sometimes unconsciously.

Unconscious bias can take two principal forms. One is often referred to as "implicit" bias. Upon confronting a member of a group which has come to be associated with negative characteristics, an individual who has internalized those associations may react differently to that person than they would to a member of their own group. This has been demonstrated repeatedly by Project Implicit, a research group based at Harvard University that has developed an online test referred to as the Implicit Association Test (IAT). When a subject connects to the test website, she or he is simultaneously shown a word and a picture of a face. Using the keys on her or his computer, the subject indicates as quickly as possible whether the word on the screen has a positive or a negative connotation. The face is changed at random from that of a white person to that of a black person. Studies of more than one million online subjects have found that white subjects in the United States consistently take a longer time to identify a word as having positive connotations when it is paired with a black face than when it is paired with a white face. Conversely, they are quicker to identify a word with negative connotations when it is paired with a black face than with a white face (Nosek et al. 2007). Subjects who demonstrate these implicit associations of white with good and black with bad will typically state that they have no personal race bias. Black subjects typically do not show this implicit association.

Another form of unconscious race bias is referred to as "stereotype bias." As described by Devine, in certain circumstances, "Automatic processes involve the unintentional or spontaneous activation of some well-learned set of associations or responses that have been developed through repeated activation in memory" (1989, p. 6). By means of example, think of a cab driver in a place like New York City driving on a busy street, hoping to get a customer. The driver sees two reasonably dressed, middle-aged men up ahead, both trying to flag him down. One is black; the other is white. Which customer does the driver pick up?

Over time the driver has become aware that, in New York City, a taxi driver's chance being robbed by a black customer is greater than by a white customer—even though the chance of either customer attempting a robbery is exceedingly small. Without thinking, and without any conscious judgment of the potential black customer, the driver picks up the white customer. The driver has internalized a stereotype that black customers are riskier than white customers and has acted on that stereotype.

In the 1990s, Danny Glover, an extremely successful black movie actor, couldn't get a cab to stop for him on the streets of Manhattan. He filed a complaint with the New York City Taxi and Limousine Commission, which sent out decoys to test Glover's assertion that cab drivers systematically passed by black customers to pick up white customers. The commission confirmed Glover's assertion and changed the law to make such biased action illegal. The cab drivers had been applying a racial stereotype, that blacks are riskier as customers than whites, to all blacks, regardless of their individual circumstances. Research has also shown that doctors, without intending to do so, may also apply negative racial stereotypes to their patients and as a consequence provide a lower level of care to black patients than white ones (van Ryn and Burke 2000; van Ryn et al. 2006).

Given that individuals might unconsciously apply negative expectations to a member of a stereotyped group, might a member of that group unconsciously apply that same stereotype to himself or herself? Recall the discussion above of the findings of Berger et al. (1977) that the status characteristics of a group can be applied to members of that group in a way that leads the group member to behave in a way that confirms that stereotype. They gave the example of teachers expecting girls to be less competent at math than boys, with the result that some girls internalize this stereotype and perform less well in math than they would have otherwise.

In 2002, Steele et al. addressed this issue in their study of undergraduate students at the University of Michigan. "In our search for answers, we soon came upon an intriguing finding: Women at the University of Michigan seemed to perform lower than their tested skills would predict in difficult math classes yet at their predicted levels in other classes that we examined such as English or, as we later found, in entry-level math classes" (p. 379). To test whether the women were responding to negative gender stereotypes, they identified a group of talented male and female undergraduates at Michigan—all with SAT scores in the top 15 percent of Michigan students, and all of whom had expressed an interest in studying math. They administered a very difficult section of the GRE math test to these students. Before giving the test, they told half of the students (selected randomly) that previous research had shown that women tended to do less well on this test than men. They told the other half of the students that men and women had been shown to perform equally well on the test. They found that "women given this instruction performed just as well as equally skilled men and significantly better than women in the stereotype-still-relevant condition of this experiment, in which participants were told that the test did show gender differences" (p. 381).

The researchers repeated this type of study with students who differed based on race (black vs. white) and documented similar effects. From this work, they defined the concept of stereotype threat in the following manner: "When a negative stereotype about a group that one is part of becomes personally relevant, usually as an interpretation of one's behavior or an experience one is having, stereotype threat is the resulting sense that one can then be judged or treated in terms of the stereotype or that one might do something that would inadvertently confirm it" (p. 389). Steele has reviewed these concepts as they apply to members of a range of potentially disadvantaged groups in his book titled *Whistling Vivaldi: And Other Clues to How Stereotypes Affect Us*. He paid particular attention to the ways in which stereotype threat can impede the academic success of students from disadvantaged racial, ethnic, or socioeconomic

groups who enter college, particularly competitive colleges and universities. When these students experience stereotype threat in addition to the sense of cultural mismatch described above for FirstGen students, their academic success can be threatened, and they are even more prone to internalizing the sense of personal inadequacy suggested by these stereotypes.

Taylor and Walton (2011), in a series of experiments with black and white university students, documented a dual impact of experiencing stereotype threat: Those students experiencing the threat not only do less well on tests of knowledge given comparable learning but are also prone to less effective patterns of learning. The researchers also showed, as in Steele's experiments, that the adverse impact of stereotype threat can be prevented by altering the context in which the tests are administered and the learning takes place.

Attribution theory: Explaining why other people act the way they do

In the mid-20th century, psychologists looked to relatively straightforward theoretical explanations of why people make the choices they do. For example, Atkinson proposed "a conception of motivation in which strength of motivation is a joint multiplicative function of motive, expectancy (subjective probability), and incentive" (1957, p. 371). How much do I want this? What are the chances I will get it if I try? What do I get in return if I succeed? These were the three questions Atkinson described people as considering when they chose whether or not to undertake a certain action.

Weiner (2010) describes how the original theory proposed by Atkinson has evolved into a more complex understanding of the factors that affect individual behavior as well as how individuals perceive the factors that affect the behavior of others around them. Under what is now commonly referred to as attribution theory, there are four principal factors that affect the outcomes of behavior: ability, effort, task difficulty, and luck. These factors can combine in different ways to affect the outcomes of specific behaviors. A key aspect of attribution theory, however, is that how the individual actor perceives the relative role of each of these factors in affecting the outcome can have powerful influences on later behavior.

Weiner describes the situation in which a student does poorly on an examination. There could be multiple reasons why this was the outcome:

- the student was not intellectually capable of passing the exam;
- the student was capable of learning the material but didn't put in sufficient effort to do so; or
- the professor was overly harsh, having given an examination that few if any students could do well on, regardless of their ability or the amount they studied for the exam.

Weiner would then add a fourth possible explanation:

- the student accidentally broke his glasses when sitting down to take the exam and couldn't read the exam questions clearly (i.e., bad luck).

The key issue is, how does the student explain this poor performance to himself or herself? How the student answers this question can affect not only future attempts at taking school exams but also the student's perception of his or her innate intellectual abilities. Recall from the discussion above that both FirstGen students and students experiencing stereotype threat tend to do less well academically than their peers from more advantaged backgrounds. These students are at risk of interpreting this poor academic performance as a reflection on

their innate abilities and as a result of expecting to do poorly again on other exams. By redefining their own abilities, they may lower their expectations for their future academic and work careers, ultimately attaining a lower socioeconomic position than they actually were capable of achieving.

Under attribution theory, individuals tend to respond differently based on two main factors: Did I do well or did I do poorly? Was the reason I did well or poorly because of something about me, or because of something external to me over which I had little control? The answers to these questions will affect how the individual reassesses his or her own abilities. "The harder the task, the more likely that success is ascribed to the self (rather than to the ease of the task) and thus the greater the pride in accomplishment" (Weiner 2010, p. 31).

If the outcome of a task is failure, the same questions arise. If a person attributes failure to causes external to herself or himself ("The test was too hard—no one could have done well" or "It was just rotten luck that I broke my glasses"), she or he is unlikely to feel responsibility for the outcome. Alternatively, she or he may simply attribute the failure to inadequate effort ("I shouldn't have stayed up so late partying the night before the exam"). However, if the outcome is failure and the individual attributes that failure to her or his own weaknesses or inadequacies, the consequences can be fundamentally different: "failure to reach a desired goal attributed to lack of aptitude is hypothesized to produce unhappiness . . . , a lowering of self-regard . . . , and shame . . . , along with a low expectation of future success and hopelessness and/or helplessness" (Weiner 2010, p. 33).

Given the cultural challenges FirstGen students and those vulnerable to stereotype threat face upon entering a competitive academic environment, it seems understandable that they would be more prone to attribute initial academic difficulties to factors within themselves (ability or effort) than to external factors (task difficulty or luck). In addition, given the relatively weak social networks many of these students experience initially, they may be unaware that other students in circumstances similar to theirs are experiencing similar difficulties. When the teaching style and attitudes of the professor put certain groups of student at a disadvantage, those students as a group are vulnerable to lower outcomes in tests or grades. For example, Moss-Racusin et al. (2012) found that science faculty from research-intensive universities exhibited a subtle bias against women in their response to written materials submitted by students. If a female student is able to discern that the disadvantage she is feeling in the science classroom affects all women in the class and not her alone, then she is less likely to attribute suboptimal academic performance to her own abilities or effort.

How, though, do we explain the actions of others within this context? If things can come out well or poorly for a variety of reasons, some having to do with factors internal to the actor and some outside the actor's control, how do we attribute the outcomes of another person's actions? It turns out that we tend to answer this question differently, based on how close a connection we have to the other person. By means of example, I will describe the reactions of a journalist to having been hit by a school bus.

René Steinke, a writer who lives in New York, wrote about the sad experience of having her old dog euthanized (2014). In what she called "a grief-stricken daze" she stepped into a Manhattan crosswalk when she saw the "Walk" sign illuminate. As she crossed the street, she did not look around her, and she did not see a school bus that was making a left turn. The bus knocked her to the ground, fortunately coming to a stop before causing her serious injury. As she recovered from her injury, she "couldn't shake the random violence of what just happened to me . . . I was appalled that the driver seemed to get off without even a ticket." From her perspective, the carelessness of the school bus driver was to blame for her injuries. If the driver had only been more careful and paid closer attention, this never would have happened.

About ten days after her injury, she received a hand-written get-well card, sent by the driver of the bus. It turns out that he was terribly upset by what had happened. Despite looking, he had not seen René crossing the street, as she had stepped into a heavily shaded section of the crosswalk. Only when he was about to hit her was he able to use the brake, barely stopping in time. He had been terrified that he might have killed her and expressed his remorse to René in the card. René had attributed the driver's actions to carelessness—a factor clearly within his control. It turned out that the accident was largely due to circumstances beyond the driver's control—the heavy shading of the crosswalk. René seems to have made what has come to be called the fundamental attribution error.

Ross (1977) has described the fundamental attribution error in the following way. When an individual reacts to a behavior he observes in someone he does not know, "his general tendency is to overestimate the importance of personal or dispositional factors relative to environmental influences . . . He jumps to hasty conclusions upon witnessing the behavior of his peers, overlooking the impact of relevant environmental factors" (p. 184). If someone does something we don't like, we assume it is probably because of a weakness or inadequacy of the person himself or herself. We tend not to consider fully environmental factors external to the person we observe that may have contributed to the outcome.

Coleman (2013) suggests that there is an additional aspect to the way we attribute outcomes to the personal characteristics of the actor as opposed to the environmental effects that are external to the actor. It depends on whether we consider the person we observe to be part of our own social network (in-group) or external to our social network. As Coleman described, "Negative acts tend to be attributed to dispositional factors more when they are performed by an out-group member than when they are performed by an in-group member. Positive acts tend to be attributed to situational factors more when they are performed by an out-group member than when they are performed by an in-group member" (p. 72). Thus, we are more likely to forgive someone we are connected to for an adverse outcome and blame someone we are not connected to for a similar outcome.

Letting the behavior of others guide our own: The bystander effect

Rather than observing the behavior of another person and coming to some conclusion as to what motivated the person to act in that manner, sometimes we turn to others around us to help us make a decision about our own behavior. If we confront an urgent problem whose outcome we could likely improve, how does the presence of others around us affect our decision of whether to intervene?

This issue came to the broad public attention in 1964. During the early morning hours, a young woman by the name of Kitty Genovese was sexually assaulted and then murdered on a street in Queens, New York. The report of the murder carried two weeks later in the *New York Times* shocked the nation: "For more than half an hour 38 respectable, law-abiding citizens in Queens watched a killer stalk and stab a woman in three separate attacks in Kew Gardens ... Not one person telephoned the police during the assault; one witness called after the woman was dead" (Gansberg 1964). How could 38 adults watching or listening out of their window allow the screams of a young woman go unheeded, with only one person acting after the victim was already dead?

Others have questioned the factual accuracy of this account, suggesting that the actual number of witnesses was substantially smaller and that the victim only died after the police arrived (Manning et al. 2007). Nonetheless, multiple people were aware that something dangerous was happening on the street near them and were likely also aware that a number of their neighbors were simultaneously witnessing the same thing. The report of this case led to a fundamental question: is the likelihood that a person will intervene in a potential emergency reduced by the awareness that others are also witnessing it?

Psychologists Bibb Latané and John Darley (1969), largely in response to the reports of the murder of Kitty Genovese and the reported failure of bystanders to intervene, conducted a series of experiments to test whether this "bystander effect" could be shown to exist in other contexts. Using university students as their test subjects, they set up a situation in which a subject would be involved in an unrelated activity when they would be exposed to one of the following situations:

- Smoke would start to billow into the room, suggesting that a fire was burning in the building.
- A tape recording would be played indicating that a large piece of furniture had fallen over on a female worker in an adjacent room, trapping her leg and possibly breaking her ankle.
- A tape recording would be played indicating that a student in another room, with whom the subject had been having a phone conversation, was apparently having an epileptic seizure and was having difficulty breathing.

In each case, based on random selection, the subject would observe these warning signs either alone or in the presence of others. The other observers were sometimes part of the experiment team who had been instructed to shrug off the warning signs and do nothing. Alternatively, they could be other research subjects involved in the same experiment. The researchers would also vary the number of other observers.

The results were consistent across these experiments. In a substantial majority of the situations, an individual who was alone would respond fairly rapidly to the emergent situation, either notifying someone else of the problem or taking direct action to help. Conversely, if the other bystanders ignored the warning and took no action, most of the study subjects would also fail to act. When the second observer in the room was not part of the research team, the study subject would tend to respond more rapidly if the subject personally knew the other observer, as compared to when the other observer was a stranger.

In the study with the smoke-filled room when the other observers were trained not to respond, only one of ten subjects reported the problem. "The other nine stayed in the waiting room as it filled up with smoke, doggedly working on their questionnaire and waving the fumes away from their faces. They coughed, rubbed their eyes, and opened the window—but they did not report the smoke" (Latané and Darley 1969, p. 251).

From these results, Latané and Darley described the "bystander effect": "When only one bystander is present in an emergency, if help is to come it must come from him . . . When there are several other observers present, however, the pressures to intervene do not focus on any one of the observers; instead the responsibility for intervention is shared among all the onlookers and is not unique to any one . . . the more bystanders who are present, the less likely any one bystander would be to intervene and provide aid" (p. 260). The presence of other bystanders who could take action seems to inhibit any one person's sense of responsibility and resulting willingness to offer help when it is needed.

Social impact theory and social loafing

If the presence of a group of bystanders reduces the propensity of an individual to intervene when help is needed, what does that suggest about the effects in general of acting alone versus acting as a member of a group? Following up on his research with Darley documenting bystander inhibition, Latané proposed a more general theory of the social impact of groups (1981). He suggested that the presence of others will influence an individual's behavioral motivation by affecting both subjective feelings and cognitive understanding. This effect, he proposed, would occur not only when the others were strangers and the behavior was to offer help or assistance but also when the others were known to the individual and the group was working collaboratively on an assigned task.

Latané had been aware of work done in the early 1900s by a French scholar named Max Ringelmann (1913). Ringelmann had hooked a large rope to a strain gauge and then asked a group of men to pull as hard as they could on the rope, first alone and then as part of a group. He found that each subject would pull hardest when he was the only puller. As the group of subjects got successively larger, the average force exerted by each worker decreased. The more an individual perceived himself to be part of a task group, with the group output measured rather than individual output, the less effort the individual would exert. Concerned that Ringelmann's findings were at least partially due to poor coordination among the pullers rather than reduced individual effort, Ingham (1974) repeated the rope-pulling study, taking steps to rule out lack of coordination as the explanation for the reduced individual output. He concluded, "The present results, then, tend to confirm the generality of the Ringelmann phenomenon—increases in group size are inversely related to individual performance" (p. 382).

Latané et al. (1979) reproduced this effect in a variety of circumstances and applied a name to the effect: social loafing. They had college students clap or cheer as loudly as they could, first alone and then as part of a group, and measured the average output volume per student, varying the circumstances in which the students interacted. In each case, students clapped or cheered more loudly as individuals than as members of a group. The researchers explained this effect in the context of Latané's social impact theory, described above, by suggesting that "whether the subject is dividing up the amount of work he thinks should be performed or whether he is dividing up the amount of reward he expects to earn with his work, he should work less hard in groups" (p. 830).

The introduction of the concept of social loafing led a number of other researchers to explore the contexts in which it will exist. Karau and Williams (1993) reviewed 78 different studies involving social loafing and found consistent evidence of its existence across tasks and groups. They identified some specific circumstances that altered the impact of social loafing. The effect was stronger when the only way to measure overall effort was at the level of the group, with no measurement of individual performance. If there was measurement at both the group and the individual level, the loafing effect was reduced somewhat. The effect was also reduced when the individual was well acquainted with the others in her or his group.

Two additional findings from their review are worth mentioning. Consistent with the interdependent/independent cultural differences described by Markus and Conner and discussed in chapter 4, Karau and Williams found that "both women and individuals in Eastern cultures are less likely to engage in social loafing, presumably because they have more group-oriented priorities than do men and individuals in Western cultures" (p. 697). Studies comparing Japanese university students with American university students confirmed that the American students would demonstrate social loafing when their task output was measured at the level of the

group as compared to the individual, whereas the Japanese students would work *harder* when their task output was measured at the level of the group rather than the individual.

Summary

We each grow up perceiving ourselves to be part of a broad social or cultural group, and as we move into adolescence and adulthood, we often become increasingly attuned to the attitudes and behaviors of those immediately around us. We tend to identify a specific group or groups to which we perceive ourselves as belonging and others to which we feel as though we don't belong. A common set of metrics we use to compare ourselves to those around us has been described as our level of capital: economic capital, cultural capital, and social capital.

Sometimes people find themselves thrown together with social groups to which they don't feel they belong. The case of the FirstGen college student attending a high-quality college or university provides an example of this situation. From studies of the experiences of First-Gen students, we have seen some of the adverse consequences that may come from this perceived mismatch as well as some of the steps that can be taken to avoid these consequences.

How one responds to an interaction with another person may also depend on how he or she explains to himself or herself that individual's motivation in undertaking the action—even if that attribution is inaccurate. How one perceives the surrounding social group can also affect how that individual responds to certain unexpected circumstances, such as another person's need for assistance. The casual bystander tends to be inhibited in responding to that need when there are others observing the same need yet failing to respond. In a similar manner, in many Western cultures, working on a task as a member of a group, rather than as an individual, will often result in exerting less effort than if one were working on the task alone. Becoming aware of the ways in which immediate social context can influence behavior is central to our overall understanding of human behavior.

REFERENCES

Appiah, K. A. 1990. Racisms. In Goldberg, D. T., ed. Anatomy of Racism, 3–17. Minneapolis: University of Minnesota Press.

Atkinson, J. W. 1957. Motivational determinants of risk-taking behavior. Psychological Review 64(6 Pt. 1): 359–72.

Berger, J., Fisek, M. H., Norman, R. Z., & Zelditch, M. Jr. 1977. Status Characteristics and Social Interaction: An Expectation-States Approach. New York: Elsevier.

Bourdieu, P. 1986. The forms of capital. In Richardson, J. G., ed. Handbook of Theory and Research for the Sociology of Education, 241–58. New York: Greenwood Press.

Coleman, M. D. 2013. Emotion and the ultimate attribution error. Current Psychology 32: 71–81.

Devine, P. G. 1989. Stereotypes and prejudice: Their automatic and controlled components. Journal of Personality and Social Psychology 56: 5–18.

Gansberg, M. 1964. 37 who saw murder didn't call police. New York Times, March 27, p. A1.

Ingham, A. G. 1974. The Ringelmann effect: Studies of group size and group performance. Journal of Experimental Social Psychology 10(4): 371–84.

Karau, S. J., & Williams, K. D. 1993. Social loafing: A meta-analytic review and theoretical integration. Journal of Personality and Social Psychology 65(4): 681–706.

Latané, B. 1981. The psychology of social impact. American Psychologist 36(4): 343–56.

Latané, B., & Darley, J. M. 1969. Bystander "apathy." American Scientist 57(2): 244–68.

Latané, B., Williams, K., & Harkins, S. 1979. Many hands make light work: The causes and consequences of social loafing. Journal of Personality and Social Psychology 37(6): 822–32.

Manning, R., Levine, M., & Collins, A. 2007. The Kitty Genovese murder and the social psychology of helping: The parable of the 38 witnesses. American Psychologist 62(6): 555–62.

Markus, H. R, & Conner, A. 2013. Clash! 8 Cultural Conflicts That Make Us Who We Are. New York: Hudson Street Press.

Moss-Racusin, C. A., Dovidio, J. F., Brescoll, V. L., Graham, M. J., & Handelsman, J. 2012. Science faculty's subtle gender biases favor male students. Proceedings of the National Academy of Sciences USA 109(41): 16474–79.

Nosek, B. A., Smyth, F. L., Hansen, J. J., et al. 2007. Pervasiveness and correlates of implicit attitudes and stereotypes. European Review of Social Psychology 18: 36–88.

Phelan, J. C., Lucas, J. W., Ridgeway, C. L., & Taylor, C. J. 2014. Stigma, status, and population health. Social Science and Medicine 103: 15–23.

Project Implicit, available at https://implicit.harvard.edu/implicit/demo, accessed 7/22/14.

Ringelmann, M. 1913. Recherches sur les moteurs animés: Travail de l'homme. Annales de l'Institut National Agronomique Series 2(12): 1–40, available at http://gallica.bnf.fr/ark:/12148/bpt6k54409695.image.f14.langEN, accessed 8/17/14.

Ross, L. 1977. The intuitive psychologist and his shortcomings: Distortions in the attribution process. Advances in Experimental Social Psychology 10: 173–220.

Steele, C. M. 2010. Whistling Vivaldi: And Other Clues to How Stereotypes Affect Us. New York: W. W. Norton.

Steele, C. M., Spencer, S. J., & Aronson, J. 2002. Contending with group image: The psychology of stereotype and social identity threat. Advances in Experimental Social Psychology 34: 379–440.

Steinke, R. 2014. 'The driver just didn't see you.' New York Times Magazine, August 8, p. 50.

Stephens, N. M., Fryberg, S. A., Markus, H. R., Johnson, C. S., & Covarrubias, R. 2012. Unseen disadvantage: How American universities' focus on independence undermines the academic performance of first-generation college students. Journal of Personality and Social Psychology 102(6): 1178–97.

Stephens, N. M., Hamedani, M. G., & Destin. M. 2014. Closing the social-class achievement gap: A difference-education intervention improves first-generation students' academic performance and all students' college transition. Psychological Science 25(4): 943–53.

Tajfel, H., & Turner, J. C. (1986). The social identity theory of intergroup behaviour. In Worchel, S., & Austin, W. G., eds. Psychology of Intergroup Relations, 7–24. Chicago, IL: Nelson-Hall.

Taylor, V. J., & Walton, G. M. 2011. Stereotype threat undermines academic learning. Personality and Social Psychology Bulletin 37(8): 1055–67.

van Ryn, M., Burgess, D., Malat, J., & Griffin, J. 2006. Physicians' perceptions of patients' social and behavioral characteristics and race disparities in treatment recommendations for men with coronary artery disease. American Journal of Public Health 96: 351–57.

van Ryn, M., & Burke, J. 2000. The effect of patient race and socio-economic status on physicians' perceptions of patients. Social Science and Medicine 50: 813-28.

Walton, G. M., & Cohen, G. L. 2011a. A brief social-belonging intervention improves academic and health outcomes of minority students. Science 331(6023): 1447-51.

———. 2011b. Sharing motivation. In Dunning, D., ed. Social Motivation, 79-101. New York: Psychology Press.

Weiner, B. The development of an attribution-based theory of motivation: A history of ideas. Educational Psychologist 45(1): 28-36.

CHAPTER 6

Motivation and Behavior

T he patterns of behavior one adopts are powerfully influenced by cultural and social context. The influence of cultural and social contexts on behavior begins in childhood
and continues throughout the transition from adolescence into
adulthood. Behavior, however, also reflects individual qualities a
child or adolescent has developed. These qualities reflect a combination of biological and psychological factors that affect the developmental process.

How early in the developmental process might key personality
and motivational traits be established such that their influence on
immediate behavior is indicative of future behavioral patterns? A
series of experiments conducted in the 1960s and 1970s by Walter
Mischel and colleagues suggests that by the age of 4, many children may have developed traits that affect their motivation when
confronted by a difficult choice—whether to eat one marshmallow now or instead to wait until a teacher says they can have two
marshmallows.

The marshmallow experiment: How long will kids wait for a treat?

In the 1960s, Walter Mischel began a now well-known experiment
to address the question of how long young children would be
willing to wait to obtain a treat. (Mischel and Ebbesen 1970;
Mischel et al. 1972) As shown in figure 6.1, the treat was a plate
with two marshmallows on it. The subjects of Mischel's study
were children who attended the Bing Preschool at Stanford University. With the parents' permission, each child was invited to
come into a room with a range of toys and other activities for the
child to play with, as well as a one-way mirror through which the
experimenters could observe the child's behavior. The teacher
explained to the child that after he or she had played alone with
the toys for a while, the teacher would come back into the room
and give the child the treat.

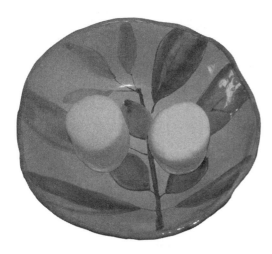

FIGURE 6.1. The Treat

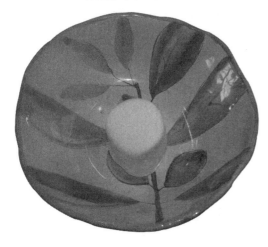

FIGURE 6.2. The Modified Treat

There was a second option, though. The teacher explained that at any time, if the child didn't want to wait for the teacher to come back, he or she could ring a bell, and the teacher would come back right away. If that happened, the child would receive a somewhat modified treat, as shown in figure 6.2—one marshmallow.

Mischel and his colleagues varied the circumstances confronting the child. For some children the plate with the marshmallows would be hidden away out of sight, while for others the plate would be on the table in plain sight. Not surprisingly, when the treat was in plain sight, it was harder for most children to wait until the teacher came back (typically about 15 minutes) in order to earn the full reward.

Would how long the child was willing and able to wait say anything about the child? Would the ability at age 4 to delay a minor gratification have any association with the choices and behaviors of that child in the future? These were the questions Mischel and colleagues reported in a follow-up study published in 1988. Between 1968 and 1974 they had included 653 children in the study. Between 1981 and 1982 they sent a follow-up questionnaire to the parents of 125 of these children, all of whom were now adolescents. Using a standardized instrument, they asked the parents to rate the child on a range of indicators. Using these parental ratings they compared children based on how long they had waited as preschoolers for their reward. The results were clear. "Specifically, children who were able to wait longer at age 4 or 5 became adolescents whose parents rated them as more academically and socially competent, verbally fluent, rational, attentive, planful, and able to deal with frustration and stress" (Mischel et al. 1988, p. 687). Mischel went on to summarize their findings: "The seconds of time preschool children were willing to delay for a preferred outcome predicted their cognitive and social competence and coping as adolescents . . . Perhaps the ability to delay gratification effectively for the sake of larger goals may itself play an increasingly powerful role in cognitive and social coping as the child matures, and . . . may be more significant for the life of the adolescent than they are for the preschool child" (pp. 692, 694).

What factors led to some children waiting for a delayed reward and others ringing the bell to obtain a smaller, yet more rapid reward? Is there some aspect of the young child's cognitive processes that made it easier for him or her to wait? Mischel and his colleagues suggested that "Although cognitive and attentional strategies and skills play an important role in the delay situation used in the present study, there is also much evidence that other factors, such as motivational and temporal considerations, expectations, and personality variables are likewise germane for a comprehensive analysis of delay of gratification" (Shoda et al. 1990, p. 985).

The role of motivation in affecting behavior

In 1968, Edwin Locke proposed what he referred to as a "Theory of Task Motivation and Incentives." Locke stated, "The basic premise of this research is that an individual's conscious ideas regulate his actions . . . The theory also views goals and intentions as mediators of the effects of incentives on task performance" (p. 157). In his proposed model, Locke described the "sequence of events leading from events in the environment to action" (p. 184). That sequence is illustrated in figure 6.3.

As described by Locke, "It appears that a necessary condition for incentives to affect behavior is that the individual recognize and evaluate the incentive and develop goals, and/or intentions in response to this evaluation" (p. 184).

Another way of describing the sequence of events Locke is referring to is to say that individuals respond to events occurring in their environment (either physical or social) first by trying to understand the event (i.e., cognition), evaluating the implications of the event for the observer, and then, based on that evaluation, deciding whether and how to act in response. As Locke suggests, an important step in the response process is setting a goal or defining an intended outcome and then taking the action necessary to attain this goal.

This perspective is quite similar to that proposed by Bandura: "The capability for self-

motivation and purposive action is rooted in cognitive activity . . . By being cognitively represented in the present, conceived future states are converted into current motivators and regulators of behavior" (1997, p. 122). We decide both whether to act and how to act based on our cognitive understanding of the goal we hope to attain, the steps necessary to attain that goal, and our ability successfully to complete those steps.

An individual's response to a given set of environmental stimuli may be affected by previous patterns of association, either positive or negative, he or she has internalized over time. In what has come to be known as "associative learning," individuals may come to associate a stimulus from the environment with an outcome that commonly follows the occurrence of that stimulus. This may happen even though the stimulus and the outcome have no causal association. The classical example of this type of conditioned response was demonstrated more than a century ago by Russian scientist Ivan Pavlov. He exposed dogs to a stimulus, such as the sound of a bell, followed shortly by the presentation of a plate of food. In what has come to be called "classical conditioning," the dogs in Pavlov's experiment would begin to salivate when they heard the bell, even though the bell was not causally connected to the appearance of the food. Humans may unconsciously develop these types of conditioned responses. For example, if a person hears a sound shortly before being suddenly frightened by something, he or she may feel a sense of fear upon hearing the sound again, even though the sound had nothing directly to do with the frightening experience.

While classical conditioning involves two causally unrelated stimuli, another form of more

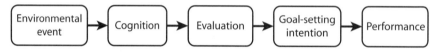

FIGURE 6.3. Locke's Model of Task Motivation

active conditioned learning involves a causal association. Referred to as "operant conditioning," this situation typically involves an action followed by an outcome that is triggered by the action. If, at the family dinner table, a child throws food she or he dislikes onto the floor, that child is likely to be punished by her or his parents, either verbally or by having some privilege withdrawn. The next time that food appears on the dinner plate, the child will, as a consequence of the punishment, be less likely to throw the food on the floor again. Conversely, a child who completes a difficult task, such as finishing a homework assignment on time, may receive a verbal or physical reward from her or his parents. Gaining a sense that the effort, if repeated, will again be rewarded may make it easier for the child to do the next day's homework assignment. Over time, the child learns that she or he can influence the outcome based on the behavior she or he adopts.

In 2002 the American Psychological Association published a volume titled *Self and Motivation* that summarized current research at that time (Tesser et al. 2002). In the introduction to the volume, the authors suggest that "the psychology of motivation raises questions about self-regulation. How do goals guide behavior?" (p. 3). They describe how some behavior is in response to goals that were set by the actor unconsciously. They go on to suggest that "More relevant to the question of motivation, however, are behaviors that reflect persistence and affect" (p. 4).

Moffitt et al. (2011) explored the role of self-regulation in the Dunedin Study, a long-term study of 1,037 children in New Zealand who were followed from the time they were three years old until they were in their mid-30s. From both direct observation as well as surveying the children's parents and preschool teachers, the researchers gauged the level of "self-control" each child exhibited. This measure included assessment of things such as impulsive aggressions, hyperactivity, lack of persistence, inattention, and impulsivity. Using this measure

they were able to determine that "children with greater self-control were more likely to have been brought up in socioeconomically advantaged families and had higher IQs" (p. 2694). They then followed these children into their adult years and found "that childhood self-control predicts physical health, substance dependence, personal finances, and criminal offending outcomes, following a gradient of self-control" (p. 2693).

How are we to understand the motivation of the preschool children in the Mischel study? Were some of them exhibiting better self-control than others? Were their motivations and behavioral responses of waiting or not waiting consciously set, or were the children responding without full conscious awareness of their motivations? How did the choice of waiting or not waiting make them feel? Did they perceive themselves as capable of persisting in their decision to await the teacher's return in order to get the two marshmallows?

Once they were adolescents, were these same motivational dynamics active in their schoolwork, in their relationships with friends, and with their families? Bandura (1997) suggested that there are three aspects to this motivational process: how we perceive the value of the goals we set for ourselves, how we understand the outcomes that are expected to occur as a consequence of certain actions, and how we attribute outcomes of our actions once we take them. I address these issues by describing the work done over more than two decades by Carrol Dweck and her colleagues.

The cognitive understanding of the self as a driver of motivation

Dweck and Legget (1988) have proposed what they describe as "A Social-Cognitive Approach to Motivation and Personality." By means of introduction, they suggest that "The task for investigators of motivation and personality is to identify major patterns of behavior and link them to underlying psychological processes" (p. 256). Based on previous work by themselves and others, they described two general patterns of behavioral responses that have been identified in both children and adults. The first of these is the "helpless" response pattern, which "is characterized by an avoidance of challenge and a deterioration of performance in the face of obstacles." The second is the "mastery-oriented" response pattern, which "involves the seeking of challenging tasks and the maintenance of effective striving under failure" (p. 256).

If some young children feel helpless in the face of a challenge, we might reasonably expect them to ring the bell early simply to gain the one marshmallow, thereby avoiding the challenge of waiting for two. By contrast, a child who enjoys challenges and continually strives to succeed even when it seems that failure may be imminent would likely wait for the teacher to return with the two marshmallows.

Dweck and Legget go on to describe how children with different perceptions of their mastery ability will set very different goals for themselves. They describe two general types of goals children may adopt: performance goals, in which children hope to have others judge them as competent based on their performance with specific tasks, and learning goals, in which children focus on increasing their competence in certain areas through continued effort, without as much consideration for specific task performance.

Dweck and Legget describe an intriguing association between the types of goals children set for themselves and their self-identity. Children who focus principally on performance goals will come to see themselves as having a fixed capacity for performance, one that can't easily be changed. Their performance on certain tasks, especially challenging tasks, will then provide a measure of their capacity. Dweck and Legget refer to this model of identity as a "fixed entity" model (p. 262).

There is a potential danger for a child who adopts a sense of one's intelligence or other capabilities as being fixed and unchangeable. A child who adopts this model and who fails to attain an expected outcome despite trying his or her best is likely to redefine his or her own capacities and abilities. With this downgraded sense of ability, the child may be less likely to take on challenges in the future, in order to avoid the risk of confirming that lack of ability through repeated failure.

By contrast, a child who has adopted the mastery model and who experiences the same level of failure to attain a given task or assignment will likely interpret this as indicating the need to continue working to improve her or his abilities, so as to succeed in the task when attempted again. As summarized by Dweck and Leggett, "the performance goal focuses the individual on judgments of ability and can set in motion cognitive and affective processes that render the individual vulnerable to maladaptive behavior patterns, whereas the learning goal creates a focus on increasing ability and sets in motion cognitive and affective processes that promote adaptive challenge seeking, persistence, and sustained performance in the face of difficulty" (p. 262).

Dweck and her colleagues performed a number of experiments testing this theoretical model. Mueller and Dweck (1998) reported on a series of six experiments in which fifth-graders were given an initial set of tasks to perform. After the students completed these tasks, the experimenters praised some of the students for their intelligence (i.e., their fixed capacity) and others for the effort they made in solving the problem (i.e., incremental learning). They then offered the children their choice of other problems sets to attempt, with some problems identified as at the same level as those first completed and some identified has harder and more challenging than the initial problems. The researchers found that those students praised for their intelligence were more likely to choose the former type of problem, thus not risking their identified intelligence, while those praised for effort were more likely to choose the latter.

A second study applied a similar approach to seventh-graders being tested on mathematical ability (Blackwell et al. 2007). The authors surveyed 373 students in public school in New York City at the time they entered seventh grade. They assessed the students' perception of intelligence as a fixed or malleable quality as well as their academic achievement record to date. Focusing on students' achievement in mathematics, they followed the students through the end of eighth grade, comparing the grades in math of students with a fixed-capacity mindset with those who had a malleable mindset. After controlling for math grades before entry into seventh grade, the malleable-mindset students had significantly higher math scores over the two-year period.

The authors also conducted an interventional experiment involving 91 students entering seventh grade, all of whom had relatively weak math scores before seventh grade. In the spring semester of seventh grade they administered a supplemental workshop to these students, with half the students getting the experimental intervention and half getting the control. As described by the authors,

> Students in both the experimental and control groups participated in similarly structured workshops, both of which included instruction in the physiology of the brain, study skills, and antistereotypic thinking. In addition, through science-based readings, activities, and discussions, students in the experimental group were taught that intelligence is malleable and can be developed; students in the control group had a lesson on memory and engaged in discussions of academic issues of personal interest to them. (p. 254)

Blackwell's research group found that, by the end of eighth grade, students in the experimental group benefited significantly from the workshop as compared to those in the control. Of the students in the experimental group,

those who had initially believed in a fixed-capacity, entity model of intelligence actually reversed the decline in math scores they otherwise would have experienced, based on the results of the first study. They began to behave more like students who initially believed in the malleable model of intelligence. From these studies, the authors concluded, "adolescents who endorse more of an incremental theory of malleable intelligence also endorse stronger learning goals, hold more positive beliefs about effort, and make fewer ability-based, 'helpless' attributions, with the result that they choose more positive, effort-based strategies in response to failure, boosting mathematical achievement over the junior high school transition" (p. 258). These results are after controlling for prior academic ability or intelligence assessment.

If children in the fifth and seventh grades have already adopted their own perception of whether their intelligence is a fixed or a malleable characteristic, how early do children learn this? Will they learn it before they get to school? Gunderson et al. (2013) addressed this question in a study of children age 1 to 3. The researchers identified a sample of 53 children in the Chicago area and started to visit each of these children in their home when the child was 14 months old. They then visited the child again every four months. During the visits they would videotape parent-child interaction for 90 minutes. They subsequently analyzed the language the parent used in conversing with the child, looking specifically at the tone and the words used when praising the child. They then categorized the frequency and type of praise exhibited by the parent, based on three categories:

1) Process praise—e.g., "you tried hard," "good job drawing," "good job trying to put that back in";
2) Person praise—e.g., "good girl/boy," "you're so smart," "you're good at that";
3) Other praise—praise that did not fall into (1) or (2) above, e.g., "Good!" or "Wow".

The researchers then recontacted the families when the children were in second or third grade (age 7 or 8) and administered a set of two surveys to assess how the children viewed intelligence and how they viewed what the authors described as "sociomoral" aspects of behavior: the extent to which children who exhibited morally acceptable behavior at age 7-8 would continue to exhibit that behavior as they grew into adolescence and adulthood. For both measures they evaluated the extent to which the children expressed a fixed capacity as compared to a malleable perception of the quality being assessed. In all their analyses the authors controlled for family income, parental education, and the child's race/ethnicity.

Overall the parents expressed process praise about as often as they expressed person praise. Also, the total amount of praise used did not differ by the gender of the child. The type of praise used, however, differed by gender, with boys hearing a higher frequency of process praise than girls (24.4% of all praise for boys vs. 10.3% of all praise for girls).

The researchers then looked at how the type of praise heard between 14 and 38 months of age was associated with the motivational framework expressed by the child at age 7 or 8. They found a significant correlation ($r=.31$, $p=.01$) between the amount of process praise heard as a young child and the child's expression of an incremental framework of both intelligence and a child's likelihood to continue to act morally over time. They then looked at gender differences at age 7-8 and found that boys were more likely than girls to express an incremental framework, a finding that holds particular significance for those studying early gender differences in math and science interest and ability. "Girls tend more than boys to attribute failures to lack of ability and thus show decreased persistence and motivation after failure. This gender difference in children's attribution styles is especially pronounced in the math and science domains, which are gender-stereotyped in favor of males" (Gunderson et al. 2013, p. 1538).

In 2007 Carol Dweck summarized the results of more than two decades of research:

> Praise is intricately connected to how students view their intelligence. Some students believe that their intellectual ability is a fixed trait. They have a certain amount of intelligence, and that's that. Students with this fixed mind-set become excessively concerned with how smart they are, seeking tasks that will prove their intelligence and avoiding ones that might not. The desire to learn takes a backseat. Other students believe that their intellectual ability is something they can develop through effort and education. They don't necessarily believe that anyone can become an Einstein or a Mozart, but they do understand that even Einstein and Mozart had to put in years of effort to become who they were. When students believe that they can develop their intelligence, they focus on doing just that. Not worrying about how smart they will appear, they take on challenges and stick to them. (p. 34)

Dweck also emphasized that the human brain is plastic, in that its underlying neural structure changes over time. Whatever aspects of a child's intellectual identity have been written into the child's cognitive sense of self can, with appropriate interventions, be rewritten over time.

If we now think again about the children in Mischel's marshmallow study, and how the ability to wait at age 4 was a significant predictor of academic and social competence in adolescence, we might then ask whether the children who rang the bell early had internalized a fixed sense of their own ability to endure a stressful situation for a period of time in order to gain a larger reward. This brings up the issue of how children, and adults, perceive time and how that perception of time affects immediate motivation to act in a certain way.

Time perspective and the *Up Series* children

In 1963, British film producer and director Michael Apted began what was to become a remarkable series of documentary films, following the lives of children in England beginning at age 7 and every seven years thereafter. This series of documentaries has come to be called the *Up Series*; the documentaries are labeled as *Seven Up, 7 Plus Seven, 21 Up,* and *28 Up,* continuing until *56 Up,* released in 2012.

Seven Up begins with an introduction by a narrator who explains that they have brought together a group of 7-year-old children "from startlingly different backgrounds." The narrator goes on to ask, "Why did we bring these children together? Because we want to catch a glimpse of England in the year 2000. The union leader and the business executive of the year 2000 are now seven years old." The narrator closes the introduction by paraphrasing a saying attributed to various Christian patriarchs: "Give me a child until he is seven, and I will give you the man."

With the many changes in British society that followed World War II, it was at that time an open question as to whether the traditional British social class system still remained intact. Would children reproduce as adults the social class into which they were born? This seemed to be the question the documentary series was intended to address. It doesn't take many episodes for us to begin to see an answer to this question. To illustrate, and to introduce a concept central to the study of motivation, I would like to introduce you to three of the children interviewed in *Seven Up:* John, Lynn, and Tony.

When we see the 7-year-old John, he is dressed in a V-neck sweater and tie and is sitting with two other boys similarly dressed. The narrator explains that John and his classmates are attending "An exclusive kindergarten school in Kensington, London." It seems apparent that they represent the upper class of British society

in the 1960s. We are also introduced to Lynn, who attends a primary school in a working-class section of the East End of London. She and her friends Jackie and Susan are often interviewed together as representing children growing up in a working-class environment. We are also introduced to Tony, who, the narrator explains, "goes to one of the older schools in London's East End slums." Tony represents a child from a lower-class background.

As part of the interview, the narrator asks each of the children what plans they have for their lives. John's reply is straightforward. "When I leave this school I'm going to College Court, and then I will be going to Westminster Boarding School if I pass the exam, and then we think I'm going to Cambridge in Trinity Hall." Lynn's response is somewhat more subdued: "I'm going to work in Woolworth's." (At the time, Woolworth's was a popular "five-and-dime" retail chain serving largely the working class.)

When the narrator asks this of Tony, we hear an immediate, enthusiastic response: "I want to be a jockey when I grow up. Yeah—I want to be a jockey when I grow up." Throughout the documentary we see 7-year-old Tony engaging in exciting yet dangerous activities—shinnying up narrow pipes, sliding down a rope dangling from a play structure, and attempting to climb over (rather than walk around) the schoolyard fence. The narrator tells us that Tony's girlfriend "calls him a monkey."

At age 7, John, Lynn, and Tony expressed very different perspectives on how they perceived the future, and the actions they were likely to take. When interviewed again at age 21, each reiterated the perspective they expressed earlier. At age 7, John saw the future in fairly clear terms. He knew what he had to do (or at least what he was expected to do) in order to attend one of the top universities in the country. At age 21 he had carried out the plan he had expressed 14 years earlier and was studying law at Oxford. (He had predicted Cambridge, but I would consider Oxford a comparable outcome.) At 7, Lynn wasn't thinking much about the future. Her attention was much more focused on the here and now, especially on her social peers. At age 21, the narrator tells us, "Lynn is now married, but still lives and works in the East End." Rather than working in Woolworth's, she is a school librarian. When it came time for her to go to what we in the United States consider as high school, she elected to attend a grammar school, which was more academically rigorous than the comprehensive school her two friends attended. Lynn got a job as a librarian, while Jackie and Susan, with their comprehensive school education, are unskilled clerical workers. When the narrator asks Lynn about her marriage, she responds, "I've been married for a year and a couple of months. You do think 'Christ, what have I done?' And I'm being honest about it. At times you think, 'Christ, what have I done?'" For Lynn, her marriage seems just to have happened.

Tony left school at age 15 to become an apprentice jockey at a riding stable. He lasted only a short while in this position. At age 21 we see him riding around London on a motorbike, trying to learn the roads so he can pass the test to become a taxi driver. The narrator asks him how many horse races he rode in during the time he was trying to become a jockey, to which Tony replies, "Only three." The narrator then asks, "Why was that?" Tony then explains his failure to become a jockey. "Obviously if I were good enough I would have had more . . . I'd have given my right arm at the time to become a jockey. I wasn't good enough—it's as easy as that."

When asked how he viewed girls and the prospect of settling down, the 21-year-old Tony said he preferred a more immediate approach to relationships. "Do you understand 4 Fs? Find 'em, feel 'em, and forget 'em. For the other F I'll let you use your own discrimination." For Tony, whether at age 7 or age 21, life seems to be about finding something exciting to do and just doing it.

At one point during the *21 Up* interviews, the narrator asks John and his upper-class friends

Andrew and Charles, "Do you think there is any truth to the ideas behind this program, that certain people have more options than others?" Charles replies, "It's certainly true that some people know they have more options, or imagine they have. I think in practical terms the difference in the number of options isn't that great. The fact is that the three of us know that there's a whole range of things we can do." Andrew follows this by suggesting, "The mere knowledge creates options itself, so I think we do have more options." John responds to Andrew's comment by saying, "I think what's undesirable is people who have had options but don't take best advantage of them."

Based on the experiences of these children from Michael Apted's documentary, we might conclude that different children, especially those from different social class backgrounds, view time and its connection to behavior differently. As a consequence, some children see a wide range of options open to them in the future, whereas others perceive a much narrower range of options. Accordingly, some children at age 7 already have a clear picture of what will likely happen in the coming years and what actions they must take to reach their envisioned goals. Others might simply take things a day at a time and let the future just happen. Still others, such as Tony, might focus on today but be more interested in seeking out something fun and exciting (perhaps even dangerous) to do.

As it turns out, most of the children first filmed in 1963 are, as middle-aged adults, exhibiting many of the same psychological traits they identified and described at age 7. "Give me a child until he is seven, and I will give you the man."

Zimbardo and time perspective

Psychologist Philip Zimbardo was one the principal authors of a study commonly known as the "Stanford Prison Experiment" (Haney et al. 1973; Zimbardo et al. 1973) in which students at

Stanford University were paid to live for one to two weeks in a closed, experimental prison environment, wherein some students were arbitrarily assigned the role of prison guard and others the role of prisoner. Within a very short time the students had taken on their respective roles with such intensity that they began to exhibit the behaviors of actual prison inmates (submissiveness) and guards (dominance and cruelty), causing the experimenters to abruptly cancel the experiment after six days. Writing more than 20 years later, Zimbardo described how that experiment clarified for him the importance of a person's perspective of time. Even though the students knew they would be returning to life as college students in a few days, they seemed to lose track of the future, instead focusing only on the present moment without consideration for the longer-term consequences of their actions. Zimbardo, who described himself as having grown up in poverty, came to the realization that, as a child, "his family and friends were prisoners of a fatalistic present. Education liberated him, and others, into a more future-oriented realm of existence" (Zimbardo and Boyd 1999, p. 1273).

Following the prison experiment, Zimbardo worked for many years to study, understand, and measure different time perspectives and their consequences. He developed a series of 56 short statements, each describing an attitude or belief (Zimbardo and Boyd 1999, p. 1287). Examples of these statements include:

- "It upsets me to be late for appointments."
- "I complete projects on time by making steady progress."
- "Fate determines much in my life."
- "I make decisions on the spur of the moment."
- "I take risks to put excitement in my life."

They then asked 606 college students, some from Stanford and some from a nearby community college, to read each statement and indicate, using a five-point scale, how characteristic the

statement was of their own perspectives and attitudes. They then conducted factor analysis of the students' responses in order to identify which of the responses tended to clump together. From this analysis they identified five groups of questions, each describing a different perspective on time. They described this analytic tool as the Zimbardo Time Perspective Inventory (ZTPI) and offered a general description of each of the five differing perspectives included in the inventory:

- Past-Negative: "Embodies a pessimistic, negative, or aversive attitude toward the past . . . associated with depression, anxiety, unhappiness, and low self-esteem";
- "Present-Hedonistic: "Orientation toward present enjoyment, pleasure, and excitement, without sacrifices today for rewards tomorrow . . . a lack of consideration of future consequences . . . low ego or impulse control";
- Future: "Characterized by planning for and achievement of future goals . . . with consideration of future consequences, conscientiousness, preference for consistency, and reward dependence, along with low levels of novelty and sensation seeking";
- Past-Positive: "Characterized by a glowing, nostalgic, positive construction of the past . . . low in depression and anxiety but high in self-esteem and happiness";
- Present-Fatalistic: "Reveals a belief that the future is predestined and uninfluenced by individual actions, whereas the present must be borne with resignation because humans are at the whimsical mercy of 'fate'" (pp. 1277-78).

In order to further validate the ZTPI scales, Zimbardo and Boyd used them in a second study involving more than 500 college students in California. They identified a number of significant correlations between the scales and an individual's personal characteristics and academic performance. Students who demonstrated a higher score on the Future perspective had higher grades in college and spent more hours per week studying. They were also less likely to exhibit aggressive tendencies or to lack impulse control. By contrast, those students who demonstrated more of a Present-Fatalistic perspective showed more aggression and more impulsive behavior, and had lower grades.

Guthrie et al. (2009) used three of the scales from the ZTPI in a series of interviews with 525 adults who were customers in a barber shop or hair salon in a suburb of Washington, DC. They wanted to see if the time perspectives exhibited were associated with level of socioeconomic attainment. The study sample was evenly split between men and women and had a diverse sampling of both racial/ethnic groups and income groups. They had each subject respond to the ZTPI prompts for three of the scales: Future, Present-Fatalistic, and Present-Hedonistic. They also asked a series of questions about subjects' occupation, income, educational level, parents' education, and current health behaviors. Subjects who had completed more formal education and who were employed in professional occupations scored higher on the Future scale and lower on the Present-Fatalistic scale than those with less education and nonprofessional occupations. The researchers also found that those whose parents had completed less formal education scored higher on the present-fatalistic scale. They found no association between subjects' present-hedonistic score and their education or occupation, nor did they find associations between any of the scales and health behaviors, after controlling for demographic variables. In summarizing their findings, the authors state, "Participants whose mother or father was less well educated had a more fatalistic time perspective, independent of their own education level. This association indicates that attitudes about fate and opportunity may be shaped in fundamental ways by childhood socioeconomic status, and that these attitudes may not be easily altered by adult experiences" (p. 2149).

Laura Carstensen has studied the role of time perspective throughout the life course as part of her "Socioemotional Selectivity Theory" (Carstensen et al. 1999). In her theory she describes the role time perspective plays in affecting motivation. "The perception of time as constrained or limited as opposed to expansive or open-ended has important implications for emotion, cognition, and motivation . . . The assessment of time plays a critical role in the ranking and execution of behaviors geared towards specific goals" (pp. 165-7).

In the *Up Series,* John, at age 7, expressed an expansive perception of time and described the series of behaviors he intended to enact in order to attain his goal of enrolling in one of England's most selective universities. Lynn, by contrast, appeared far more fatalistic as to what time held for her. When asked about her future, she said she would be working in Woolworth's, without any clear idea how she would get there. When, at age 21, she looked back over her life, her response was, "Christ, what have I done?" At age 7, Tony had little if any concept of the future other than that he wanted to be a jockey. He abandoned school in an attempt to become a jockey but as an apprentice lasted only three rides. "I wasn't good enough—it's as easy as that." Tony seems to match fairly well Zimbardo's concept of the Present-Hedonistic perspective. Consistent with the findings above of the study by Guthrie et al., Tony and Lynn had working-class parents, presumably poorly educated, while John clearly had well-educated parents. The time perspectives they observed in their own parents, coupled with the time perspectives they expressed and enacted as children and adolescents, were strongly associated with their socioeconomic position as young adults. "Give me a child until he is seven, and I will give you the man."

Noncognitive aspects of motivation and Maslow's hierarchy of needs

Until now we have been looking at motivation principally as a combination of cognitive perceptions and personality traits. What about when we are motivated to act based on physiological needs rather than cognitive perceptions? When we perceive hunger, we perceive a powerful motivation to eat. This motivation, however, is coming from a series of peptide molecules that communicate between the stomach and the hypothalamus. Similarly, the motivation to find warmth in the face of excessive cold comes through chemical and neurological messages generated by our thermostatic control mechanism in the hypothalamus. How do we relate these basic needs to the more cognitively derived motivation involved in deciding whether to ring the bell or wait for the teacher to return with two marshmallows?

As early as 1943, psychologist Abraham Maslow offered a theory to relate these motivational factors. He identified a range of needs that humans seek to fulfill but do so in a hierarchical manner. "Human needs arrange themselves in hierarchies of pre-potency. That is to say, the appearance of one need usually rests on the prior satisfaction of another, more pre-potent need" (p. 370).

Maslow described a series of five basic needs. The first of these are physiological needs necessary to maintain homeostasis within the body. These include the need for basic nutrients and the need to maintain a constant body temperature. These needs, according to Maslow, are the most fundamental, as a person lacking both food and some of the higher needs "would probably hunger for food more strongly than for anything else" (p. 373).

Once one has satisfied the need for food and warmth, at least above a certain threshold, one's attention then turns to addressing the need for safety. Infants in particular are acutely aware of a perceived lack of safety, though the need for safety is present for adults as well. Once the needs for food and for safety have been met, Maslow identifies social needs for love and belonging as the next most important. "If both the physiological and the safety needs are fairly well gratified, then there will emerge the love and affection and belongingness needs, and the whole cycle already described will repeat itself with this new center" (p. 381). The need to belong encompasses both an intimate, trusting relationship with another person and belonging to a broader social group, such as a social or religious group.

Maslow then raises an interesting point—is the perceived need for sexual intimacy a physiological need, a need for connectedness, or both? Much in the same way that psychologist Erik Erikson (discussed in chapter 7) suggested that sexual attraction transitions from being part of one's identity as an adolescent to expressing a young adult's need to form intimate, loving relationships with others, Maslow attributes both physiological and social belonging aspects to the perceived sexual need.

If one has satisfactorily addressed physiological needs, the need for safety, and the need for social belonging, the next requirement Maslow identifies is that "for self-respect, or self-esteem, and for the esteem of others" (p. 381). This self-esteem includes both a sense of achievement and a sense of independence and freedom. Once this need has been met, Maslow then describes the highest of the needs: that for self-actualization. "Even if all these needs are satisfied, we may still often (if not always) expect that a new discontent and restlessness will soon develop, unless the individual is doing what he is fitted for . . . What a man *can* be, he *must* be" (p. 382).

As shown in figure 6.4, the traditional way to display Maslow's hierarchy graphically is as a triangle, with the more basic motivational needs on the bottom and the higher needs above. This configuration suggests that the physiological and safety needs are of greater import than the needs for self-esteem and self-actualization, as they

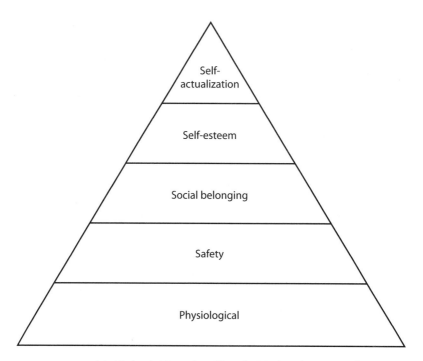

FIGURE 6.4. Maslow's Hierarchy of Needs, Displayed as a Triangle

form the foundation on which the self is constructed. The clear delineation between the levels in this model also seem to suggest that a more basic need must be fully satisfied before energy or attention can be paid to the need above. Maslow actually contradicts this perception in his original work. "This statement might give the false impression that a need must be satisfied 100 per cent before the next need emerges. In actual fact, most members of our society who are normal, are partially satisfied in their basic needs and partially unsatisfied in all their basic needs at the same time. A more realistic description of the hierarchy would be in terms of decreasing percentages of satisfaction as we go up the hierarchy of prepotency" (p. 388). This perspective is illustrated in figure 6.5, in which the rectangles, each of the same size, are layered sequentially on each other, while the gray area within the rectangle indicates the extent to which that need has been met.

One thus does not need to satisfy fully the needs of hunger and safety in order to seek out social belonging. Similarly, one who lacks a partner or social group can still seek out self-actualization and self-esteem. Many have pointed out that certain individuals actually eschew food, warmth, or safety in order to work toward goals that, once attained, will provide them with a deep sense of actualization.

As he wrote increasingly about the implications of his theory, Maslow eventually added additional needs to this list. In a book first published in 1954, Maslow identified "the desires to know and to understand" and "the aesthetic needs" as also important for a full life: "The needs for order, for symmetry, for closure, for completion of the act, for system, and for structure" (1987, p. 26). In a 1970 essay, Maslow identified one additional human need: that for transcendence. As Maslow got closer to his own death, he recognized that "Man has a higher and transcendent nature, and this is part of his essence" (Maslow 1970, p. xvi). Maslow described this need as consistent with traditional religious teachings of accepting a higher order to life and

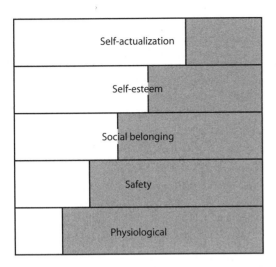

FIGURE 6.5. Maslow's Hierarchy of Needs, Displayed as a Rectangle

experiencing a heightened awareness of this order, often through helping others to meet their own needs. It is interesting to compare Maslow's need for transcendence identified toward the end of his life with the ninth stage of development described by Erikson Erikson's widow, Joan, only after Erik had died (see chapter 7). Our understanding of the world and our place in it may change as we come closer to the end of our time here, something experienced both by leading psychologists and by those of us who are not.

Tay and Diener (2011) evaluated data from a poll conducted globally that included subjects in 123 countries. They assessed the extent to which respondents' needs were met, based on Maslow's hierarchy of needs, and examined subjects' evaluation of their subjective well-being. They did identify a significant association between need fulfillment and well-being but noted that the hierarchical sequence identified by Maslow was not consistently supported by evidence. For example, "people in impoverished nations, with only modest control over whether their basic needs are fulfilled, can nevertheless find a measure of well-being through social relationships and other psychological needs over which they have more control" (p. 364).

One final conclusion reached by Tay and Diener was that living in a society in which those around us have had their basic needs met was associated with an increased sense of well-being, independent of an individual's own level of need fulfillment. In the process of addressing our own needs, we are also consistently aware of the needs of those around us, especially those with whom we form close social connections. The social and cultural context in which we live and grow up can affect our sense of well-being as well as our capacity to meet our own personal needs.

Summary

As they move through childhood and adolescence, individuals develop, to a greater or lesser degree, a sense of their own ability to influence the things that happen to them. Based on this perception of their ability to affect future outcomes, they may become capable of setting longer-term goals for things they want to achieve and of taking the actions necessary to attain those goals. Factors in their immediate environment can have powerful effects on how children develop and subsequently act on these motivations. Some children will come to view themselves as having an innately fixed capacity at achieving certain outcomes, while others may develop a sense that they can increase that capacity through additional effort. Some children will come to focus mostly on the present, paying relatively little attention to the longer-term consequences of behaviors undertaken today. Other children may develop a substantially clearer concept of the future and their ability to affect future outcomes.

These aspects of motivation that begin to develop during childhood can have long-term impacts on subsequent behavior as adolescents and as adults and on the extent to which an individual is capable of fulfilling his or her basic needs, whether they be the need for food, shelter, and safety or higher-level needs for a sense of social belonging and self-esteem. All of these factors can have lifelong effects on the overall level of attainment one realizes and the level of well-being one experiences. The motivational patterns one develops over time will be strongly influenced by the broader social and cultural context in which one grows up and lives.

Many of the motivational theorists cited above suggest that motivation is closely linked with the personality traits an individual develops. While motivation and personality certainly overlap, there are other aspects of personality that go beyond specific task motivation, influencing how one relates to others as well as how one perceives himself or herself. The next chapter introduces us to many of the core personality theorists and theories that have added substantially to our understanding of behavior.

REFERENCES

Bandura, A. 1997. Self-Efficacy: The Exercise of Control. New York: W. H. Freeman and Company.

Blackwell, L. S., Trzesniewski, K. H., & Dweck, C. S. 2007. Implicit theories of intelligence predict achievement across an adolescent transition: A longitudinal study and an intervention. Child Development 78(1): 246-63.

Carstensen, L. L., Isaacowitz, D. M., & Charles, S. T. 1999. Taking time seriously: A theory of socioemotional selectivity. American Psychologist 54(3): 165-81.

Dweck, C. S. 2007. The perils and promises of praise. Educational Leadership 65(2): 34-39.

Dweck, C. S., & Leggett, E. L. 1988. A social-cognitive approach to motivation and personality. Psychological Review 95(2): 256-73.

Gunderson, E. A., Gripshover, S. J., Romero, C., et al. 2013. Parent praise to 1- to 3-year-olds predicts children's motivational frameworks 5 years later. Child Development 84(5): 1526-41.

Guthrie, L. C., Butler, S. C., Ward, M. M. 2009. Time perspective and socioeconomic status: A link to socioeconomic disparities in health? Social Science and Medicine 68(12): 2145-51.

Haney, C., Banks, W. C., & Zimbardo, P. G. 1973. A study of prisoners and guards in a simulated prison. Naval Research Review 30: 4-17.

Locke, E. M. 1968. Toward a theory of task motivation and incentives. Organizational Behavior and Human Performance 3: 157-89.

Maslow, A. H. 1943. A theory of human motivation. Psychological Review 50(4): 370-96.

———. 1970. Religions, Values, and Peak Experiences. New York: Penguin.

———. 1987. Motivation and Personality. 3rd edition. New York: Harper and Row.

Mischel, W., & Ebbesen, E. B. 1970. Attention in delay of gratification. Journal of Personality and Social Psychology 16(2): 329-37.

Mischel, W., Ebbesen, E. B., & Zeiss, A. R. 1972. Cognitive and attentional mechanisms in delay of gratification. Journal of Personality and Social Psychology 21(2): 204-18.

Mischel, W., Shoda, Y., & Peake, P. K. 1988. The nature of adolescent competencies predicted by preschool delay of gratification. Journal of Personality and Social Psychology 54(4): 687-96.

Moffitt, T. E., Arseneault, L., & Belsky, D. 2011. A gradient of childhood self-control predicts health, wealth, and public safety. Proceedings of the National Academy of Sciences 108(7): 2693-98.

Mueller, A. M., & Dweck, C. S. 1998. Praise for intelligence can undermine children's motivation and performance. Journal of Personality and Social Psychology 75(1): 33-52.

Shoda, Y., Mischel, W., & Peake, P. K. 1990. Predicting adolescent cognitive and self-regulatory competencies from preschool delay of gratification: Identifying diagnostic conditions. Developmental Psychology 26(6): 978-86.

Tay, L., & Diener, E. 2011. Needs and subjective well-being around the world. Journal of Personality and Social Psychology 101(2): 354-65.

Tesser, A., Stapel, D. A., & Wood, J. V., Eds. 2002. Self and Motivation. Washington, DC: American Psychological Association.

Zimbardo, P. G., & Boyd, J. N. 1999. Putting time in perspective: A valid, reliable individual-differences metric. Journal of Personality and Social Psychology 77: 1271-88.

Zimbardo, P. G., Haney, C., Banks, W. C., & Jaffe, D. 1973. The mind is a formidable jailer: A Pirandellian prison. New York Times Magazine, April 8, p. 36.

CHAPTER

7

Personality, Behavior, and Well-Being

Personality traits and patterns of motivation are often closely linked, and these characteristics and the linkages between them begin to develop early in childhood. Both personality and motivation can affect the behaviors children begin to adopt as they grow into childhood and adolescence.

In 2012, journalist and author Paul Tough published a book that described his extensive exploration into the question of how children succeed. In his introduction to the book, Tough asks the central questions he hopes to address: "Who succeeds and who fails? Why do some children thrive while others lose their way?" (p. xxiv). In his conclusion, he offers an answer to these questions: "Science suggests . . . that the character strengths that matter so much to young peoples' success are not innate; they don't appear in us magically, as a result of good luck or good genes. And they are not simply a choice. They are rooted in brain chemistry, and they are molded, in measureable and predictable ways, by the environment in which children grow up" (p. 196).

Children's learned behavioral patterns develop through repetitive interaction with their social and cultural environment and the neurological coding of these experiences (see chapter 8). Concurrently with developing their cognitive awareness of the world and its behavioral expectations, children also develop a sense of self. Early in the developmental process, this sense of self begins to become increasingly differentiated from the people and things children observe and interact with.

The American Psychological Association defines the concept of personality as "The unique psychological qualities of an individual that influence a variety of characteristic behavior patterns (both overt and covert) across different situations and over time." Thus who we are—our personality—will be reflected in how we act under various circumstances.

Who we are, as reflected in our perceptions and behaviors, changes substantially from birth through childhood and into adolescence and young adulthood. We are not born with our personality set in place. Rather, it changes and evolves as we grow and experience new things. Two 20th-century authors in particular have described the process of the development of personality as occurring in distinct stages, beginning at birth. While these descriptions of the stages of personality development share much in common, the models of personality development proposed by Sigmund Freud and Erik Erikson also differ in a number of key ways.

Sigmund Freud and the stages of psychosexual development

Sigmund Freud was born in 1856 in what was then called Moravia, a region that is now part of the Czech Republic. When he was about 4 his family moved to Vienna, where he grew up, experiencing the anti-Semitism that was then prevalent in much of Europe. He did well in school and entered the University of Vienna when he was 17, electing to study medicine. He finished his medical training in 1881 and embarked on a career in research, with an early interest in diseases of the brain and nervous system.

After spending about five years working in a hospital, Freud left and opened a private clinical practice that focused on treating patients with various nervous conditions. As this practice progressed, Freud began to develop his own theories of why these adult nervous conditions occurred and what might be done to treat them. He published these theories in two books: *The Interpretation of Dreams* in 1900 and *Three Essays on the Theory of Sexuality* in 1905. I will focus on the latter book.

Even though he rarely treated children, Freud came to have an understanding of the childhood origins of many of the different nervous conditions he observed in his patients. He also interpreted many of these conditions as having an abnormality of sexual behavior at their centers. He thus based his theory on factors that could impair the normal sexual development of children.

Freud saw human infants as possessing sexual instincts from birth and suggested that a tendency to what he referred to as "perversions" of these instincts was a normal part of childhood development. As described in the summary to his 1905 book, "a disposition to perversions is an original and universal disposition of the human sexual instinct and that normal sexual behavior is developed out of it as a result of organic changes and psychical inhibitions occurring in the course of maturation" (p. 97). Those who, for some reason pertaining to the circumstances of their development as children, are unable to adapt to the changing nature of their sexual feelings are as adults prone to develop what Freud referred to as "neurosis." As Freud describes, "A formula begins to take shape which lays it down that the sexuality of neurotics has remained in, or been brought back to, an infantile state" (1905, p. 38). It then becomes the psychoanalyst's job to help the patient revisit the period of childhood sexuality that was never fully resolved.

A central principle of Freud's theory about the sexual instincts of children is the concept of erotic pleasure. The *Oxford English Dictionary* defines "erotic" as "pertaining to the passion of love." What does a newborn infant "love"? At first, she loves to suck at her mother's breast, both for the nutritional value of the breast milk and for the intense sense of pleasure she gets from feeling the nipple in her mouth. This sense of pleasure is key to what Freud considers as "sexual." The sensations generated in the nerves of the infant's lips and tongue trigger a positive emotional sensation in the amygdala, a key cortical area of the brain that plays a central role in sensing and responding to emotion. After repeated experiences of nursing at her mother's breast, the newborn infant is likely to develop a form of memory of these sensations. As part of the normal response to such sensations, the infant will seek them out again. As the infant grows somewhat older and no longer needs to rely on breast milk to the same extent for providing nutrition, she may derive intense pleasure from sucking on her thumb or a pacifier, thereby restimulating the nerves in the mouth that were originally stimulated by sucking at the mother's breast.

Freud applies two terms to this stepwise development of the infant's response to stimulation of the mouth. He refers to the instinctual sensing of pleasure and associated desire for repeated sensing of that pleasure as occurring in the *id*. As the infant becomes more conscious of her ability to find that pleasure from sources other than the mother's breast and adapts to the necessity of delayed gratification, Freud describes the infant's *ego* as assuming more control. As the child develops more awareness of his or her familial and social surroundings, he or she also develops a higher level of self-awareness, identified by Freud as the *superego*. As described by Fleming, "The superego develops in the child as it becomes aware of rights and wrongs. It is in part an internal moral compass or conscience" (2004b, p. 8-19).

Many people would not consider this pleasure-seeking behavior on the part of an infant to be a form of sexuality. Nonetheless, Freud uses this term to describe the fixation on seeking oral pleasure commonly seen in infants. He describes the infant's mouth and lips as an "erotogenic zone," in that they provide pleasure when stimulated. He also identifies two other erotogenic zones from which the developing child seeks pleasure at different stages in the development process: the anal canal and the genitals.

As awareness of and control over bowel function increases, at about the age of 2 the child's attention begins to focus on the sensations generated in the anus. As Steven Marcus describes in his introduction to Freud's book,

"The anal zone is the second area of erotogenic pleasure. The sexual excitement of this zone are both active and passive and involve both the stimulation of the mucous membranes and the control (and release) of the sphincter muscle" (1905, p. xxxv). As the child begins to differentiate himself from others in the world and to seek more control over his environment, being able to take control over the sensations emanating from the anal area becomes more important.

Between the ages of 3 and 6, a developmental stage Freud refers to as the phallic stage, the child's focus shifts from the anal area to the sensations generated in the genitals. "It is not until a third phase has been reached that the genital zones proper contribute their share in determining sexual life, and in children this last phase is developed only so far as to a primacy of the phallus" (p. 99). These genital sensations include both the sensation of urination and bladder control and of touching the genitals directly.

From about the age of 6 until puberty, the developing child occupies a stage of latency, suppressing the desire for erotogenic stimulation, largely in response to social norms and parental restrictions. During these years the child redirects her or his energies and attentions to growth-related activities, such as learning in school, developing social skills, and interacting with social networks outside the family. Once the sex hormones generated during and after puberty began to exert their effect, both through the development of secondary sex characteristics in the body and the growing awareness of sexual attraction to others, the growing child enters the genital stage, the last stage described by Freud. It is during this stage that what we now commonly view as sexual activity begins, with exploration of either heterosexual or homosexual interaction, the seeking of sexual partners, and the desire to have children.

In chapter 9 I will address the issue of cognition as distinct from personality. While

TABLE 7.1. Comparison of Piaget's Stages of Cognitive Development with Freud's Stages of Psychosexual Development

Piaget			Freud		
Stage	Age	Development of cognitive characteristics	Stage	Age	Development of psychosexual characteristics
Sensory-motor	Birth–2	Sense of self, beginning of language	Oral	Birth–2	Focus on sensations from nursing/sucking
Preoperational	2–7	Symbolic meanings, expanded language, understands numbers	Anal	2–3	Focus on anal sensations and bowel control
			Phallic	3–6	Focus on genital sensations and bladder control
Concrete operational	7–12	Classification of objects, logical reasoning, mathematical ability	Latent	6–puberty	Focus on educational and social development
Formal operational	12 and older	Hypothetical reasoning, abstract relationships, moral concepts	Genital	Puberty–adult	Sexual attraction, sexual activity, partnership, childbearing

personality reflects our image of our self, cognition reflects how we think and what we know and is based largely on the neurobiological storage of memories and associations. As I discuss in more detail in chapter 9, Jean Piaget, a Swiss developmental psychologist, described the stepwise development in cognitive ability that parallels the development of the brain's neural capacities. Before looking at the various psychological impacts Freud describes as caused by adverse experiences during these phases of psychosexual development, it will first be informative to compare the stages of personality development described by Freud to the stages of cognitive development described by Piaget. Table 7.1 compares these stages of development.

We can see a striking similarity in the development stages as described by these two psychological theorists. Freud divides the years from 2 until about 6 or 7 into two stages, whereas Piaget treats this as a single stage. Otherwise the stages of development are nearly identical. Another similarity is the perception of both au-

thors that the human brain has certain capabilities at birth and can only develop further capabilities as it grows and develops. As described above, Freud thought that "normal sexual behavior developed . . . as a result of organic changes and psychical inhibitions occurring during the course of maturation" (p. 97). This view is quite similar to that of Piaget, that a combination of neural development and social learning enables the growing child to acquire successively more complex forms of cognitive ability.

Thus far I have described the normal stages of psychosexual development as characterized by Freud. I should emphasize that Freud delineated these stages so as to understand better the abnormal psychological states he encountered in his adult patients. From Freud's perspective, adult behavioral neuroses often originate in unresolved conflicts stemming from the earlier stages of development during childhood. For example, a child may never have fully adjusted to the role either the same-sex parent or the opposite-sex parent plays in affecting the child's developing awareness. Especially if the child experiences traumatic events involving a parent during these early formative years, the child may repress these feelings rather than deal with them. As described by Fleming, "For Freud repression was the most important of many defense mechanisms that protect people from being overwhelmed with anxiety. But a price is paid for failing to recognize unconscious feelings and impulses, as repressing them can lead to neurosis, or psychological maladjustment" (2004b, p. 8-13). The psychoanalyst's job, as seen by Freud, was to help the patient let go of these repressed emotions in order to reduce the adverse impact of the neurosis associated with them.

In the final paragraph of his *Three Essays on the Theory of Sexuality,* Freud closes his summary of these issues with what is, from today's perspective, a fascinating observation: "The unsatisfactory conclusion, however, that emerges from these investigations of the disturbances of sexual life is that we know far too little of the biological processes constituting the essence of sexuality to be able to construct from our fragmentary information a theory adequate to the understanding alike of normal and pathological conditions" (1905, p. 109). Freud seemed to appreciate the rudimentary level of scientific knowledge at the turn of the 20th century regarding the biological mechanisms underlying brain structure and function. He also seemed to suggest that a more detailed knowledge of neurobiology might someday extend the theories he proposed.

Erik Erikson and the stages of psychosocial development

Erik Erikson had a difficult and complex childhood. He was born in Germany in 1902, the child of an unmarried Jewish woman and a father believed to be Danish. His mother married another man when Erikson was 3, "but because of these unusual circumstances, he had an 'identity problem,' which surely influenced

not only his unconventional lifestyle, but also his ideas about the crises that each person encounters at each stage of his or her life" (Fleming 2004a, p. 9-1). Erikson first moved to Vienna to teach art to the children of Americans who were studying psychoanalysis under Freud. Soon he began to study psychoanalysis himself, working with Freud's daughter Anna and focusing on child psychiatry. He subsequently moved to the United States, where he held a range of academic positions. He ultimately moved to work at the Austen Riggs mental health treatment center in Massachusetts in 1951.

By the time he joined Austen Riggs, Erikson had developed his own theory of the normal course of psychological development of children and how difficulties encountered during the development process could affect the personality and behavior of adults. He first published these theories in 1950 in a book titled *Childhood and Society.* While certainly based on Freud's theory, Erikson's views differed in a number of ways from those of Freud.

- Erikson did not see sexual feelings as playing a central role in the psychological development of children.
- Erikson saw a major role for the social and cultural context in which a child grows up in affecting the various stages of development.
- Erikson placed less importance on the conscious/unconscious nature of childhood development as represented by Freud's ego/id categories.
- As compared to the five stages Freud described, Erikson described eight distinct stages of development, beginning at birth and continuing through old age and death. As shown in table 7.2, he referred to these as "The Eight Ages of Man."

At each of these developmental stages, Erikson described the individual as confronting a crisis. For example, in the first stage, from birth through approximately 18 months of age, an

TABLE 7.2. The Eight Ages of Man as Described by Erik Erikson (1950)

Stage	Approximate age	Crisis confronted	Virtue to be attained
1	Birth–18 months	Basic trust vs. basic mistrust	Hope
2	2–3 years	Autonomy vs. shame and doubt	Will
3	4–6 years	Initiative vs. guilt	Purpose
4	7–12 years	Industry vs. inferiority	Competence
5	13–19 years	Identity vs. role confusion	Fidelity
6	20–34 years	Intimacy vs. isolation	Love
7	35–64 years	Generativity vs. stagnation	Care
8	~65 years to death	Ego integrity vs. despair	Wisdom

infant either comes to trust or to mistrust his caregiver (usually the mother). It is normal for the child to experience periods of each. Even in a close and supportive relationship, the mother can't be present at every moment the child wishes her there. Over time, though, the child will come to trust that the mother will return and will be there if really needed. This will allow the child to resolve this crisis and to come out of this stage with a sense of hope, a feeling that, even if difficulties are confronted in the future, things will turn out well. If, on the other hand, the child finds the sense of mistrust coming to predominate, the child may come out of that stage with a strong sense of mistrust in others and experience feelings of insecurity in the future.

In this same way, Erikson described a core conflict to be confronted at each developmental stage and a strength or virtue to be obtained through successful resolution of the conflict. For example, between ages 4 and 6, as the child becomes increasingly aware of the social and cultural context in which he or she is growing up, he or she will need to address the conflict between wanting to take the initiative in choosing how to act and feeling guilty if a parent or other person of authority sees the child's action as inappropriate. A successful resolution of this conflict can result in the child developing a

sense of purpose and the confidence to act according to his or her own sense of self. Inadequate resolution can result in a feeling of being inhibited in one's actions.

As seen by Erikson, the unsuccessful resolution of any of these crises can result in feelings of anxiety that can affect one's psychological health throughout life. As described by Erikson, "Anxieties are diffuse states of tension . . . which magnify and even cause the illusion of an outer danger, without pointing to appropriate avenues of defense or mastery" (1950, p. 406). These anxieties can be so powerful as to impair normal human interaction. It then becomes the therapist's job, as seen by Erikson, to help the affected adult identify the earlier unresolved conflict that caused the anxiety, often by revisiting childhood experiences, and to gain resolution through a deeper understanding of the factors that originally prevented successful resolution.

It is interesting to look at the conflicts faced by older adults and the potential consequences of failing to resolve these conflicts. For example, as one grows beyond age 65 and either retires from or plans to retire from one's lifetime of work, it is normal to look back and ask, "How did I do? Did I do a good job with my life? Did I act with integrity? Was my life worthwhile?" Successful resolution of this crisis can help one to move into the older years with a sense of wisdom and a life well lived. By contrast, failure to resolve this can lead to a sense of failure and despair.

Erik Erikson died in 1994 at the age of 91. In 1997, Joan Erikson, Erik's wife of 64 years, wrote a preface for an extended edition of a book she and Erik coauthored earlier, titled *The Life Cycle Completed: Extended Version with New Chapters on the Ninth Stage of Development*. Joan Erikson describes both her and Erik's slow decline as they passed through their eighties and entered their nineties.

> Although at eighty we began to acknowledge our elderly status, I believe we never faced its challenges realistically until we were close to ninety . . . At ninety we woke up in foreign territory . . . As we passed through the years of generativity, it had never felt as though the end of the road were here and now. We had still taken years for granted. At ninety the vistas changed; the view ahead became limited and unclear. Death's door, which we always knew was expectable but had taken in stride, now seemed just down the block. (p. 4)

Joan Erikson died in 1997, the year she described the Ninth Stage of Man.

Criticisms of the Freud/Piaget/ Erikson perspectives on the stages of development

While Freud's theory of psychosexual development, Erikson's theory of psychosocial development, and Piaget's theory of cognitive development have come to be core foundational elements in our understanding of human psychological development, not everyone agrees with or supports their perspectives. One of the principal faults attributed to these theorists is their consistent focus on the male perspective, assuming that the development of females will then follow in suit, albeit with some modifica-

tion based on sexual differences. Take for example Freud's phallic stage, in which the boy between the ages of 3 and 6 becomes increasingly aware of his penis and comes to enjoy feeling and touching it. Freud seems to assume that girls will develop the same awareness of and pleasure from their clitoris, seen by Freud as the female equivalent of the penis.

Another example of gender bias is often described in Erikson's fifth stage, occurring during adolescence, in which the teenager seeks to resolve the conflict between identity and role confusion in order to gain a clear sense of individual identity. In a preface to the a reissue of a book she originally published in 1982, psychologist Carol Gilligan (1993) describes her work at the Harvard Project on Women's Psychology and the Development of Girls. Gilligan received her doctorate in psychology in 1964 from Harvard University. In 1967 she began teaching at Harvard, and while there she worked with both Erik Erikson and Lawrence Kohlberg, a developmental psychologist who described a theory of moral development.

Gilligan raised fundamental questions about Kohlberg, Erikson's, and Freud's work, writing, "my questions are about psychological processes and theory, particularly theories in which men's experience stands for all of human experience—theories which eclipse the lives of women and shut out women's voices . . . When I was working with Erik Erikson and Lawrence Kohlberg at Harvard, teaching psychology in the tradition of Freud and Piaget, I remember moments in classes when a woman would ask a question that illuminated with sudden brilliance the foundations of the subject we were discussing" (p. xiii-xiv).

Gilligan stated explicitly how she viewed the psychological development of women as differing fundamentally from that of men. "I introduce a relational voice and develop its counterpoint with traditional ways of speaking about self, relationship, and morality . . . I reframe women's psychological development as centering on a struggle for connection rather than speaking about women in the way that psychologists have spoken about women—as having a problem in achieving separation" (p. xv).

Gilligan also speaks critically of the traditional (male) discussion of the developmental dichotomy of nature vs. nurture. "At its most troubling, the present reduction of psychology either to sociology or biology or some combination of the two prepares the way . . . for the suffocation of voice and the deadening of language" (p. xix). The voice that women bring to their relationships with others reflects an inseparable combination of female biology and the female experience. "Clearly, these differences arise in a social context where factors of social status and power combine with reproductive biology to shape the experiences of males and females and the relations between the sexes" (p. 20). Gilligan describes the psychological development of girls and women not as creating a crisis of individual identity but rather as "a progression of relationships towards a maturity of interdependence" (p. 155).

Understanding adult personality traits using the "Big Five"

So far in this chapter we have been discussing different theories on the development personality as part of the growth and maturation process, all of which point to a common conclusion. By the time they reach adulthood, individuals have developed various personality traits, some positive and some less so, based on their experiences throughout childhood. Is there a way to examine the patterns of personality characteristics present in adults, regardless of their source, so as better to understand how personality is expressed as behavior?

Beginning in the mid-20th century, psychologists began applying what has been described as a "lexical" approach to answering this question, defined by the *Oxford English Dictionary* as "pertaining or relating to the words or vocabulary of a language." John and Srivastava (1999) described the initial attempts by Allport and Odbert (1936) to identify all the words in the dictionary that could be used to describe personality and behavioral characteristics. They came up with a list of nearly 18,000 words and immediately recognized that simply listing the words was not useful. Beginning in the 1940s, Cattell worked over a period of several decades to simplify the list of words used as personality descriptors, suggesting that a much smaller set of words could be divided into sixteen categories of personality traits. (Cattell et al. 1970). Norman (1967) subsequently suggested that an even smaller set of personality descriptors could be grouped into seven categories.

As described by John and Srivastava, the categories of words identified by Allport and Odbert and by Norman "overlap and have fuzzy boundaries, leading some researchers to conclude that distinctions between classes of personality descriptors are arbitrary and should be abolished" (p. 104). While many psychologists abandoned the effort to develop a standardized list of personality traits, others continued to work on this issue. Fortunately they were helped substantially by the growing use of computers in the 1970s and 1980s to perform complex mathematical and statistical tasks. Using a method referred to as factor analysis, it was possible to group various words used in describing personality into five broad categories. By the 1980s there was a growing consensus that these categories, described as the "Big Five Factor Structure" (Goldberg 1990) were valid from a research perspective. As summarized by John and Srivastava, "After decades of research, the field is finally approaching consensus on a general taxonomy of personality traits, the 'Big Five' personality dimensions" (p. 103). They go on, however, to qualify somewhat how the Big Five are best understood, suggesting that "the Big Five structure does not imply that personality differences can be reduced to only five traits.

TABLE 7.3. The Big Five Personality Traits

Extraversion implies an energetic approach to the social and material world and includes traits such as sociability, activity, assertiveness, and positive emotionality.

Agreeableness contrasts a prosocial and communal orientation toward others with antagonism and includes traits such as altruism, tender-mindedness, trust, and modesty.

Conscientiousness describes socially prescribed impulse control that facilitates task- and goal-directed behavior, such as thinking before acting, delaying gratification, following norms and rules, and planning, organizing, and prioritizing tasks.

Neuroticism contrasts emotional stability and even-temperedness with negative emotionality such as feeling anxious, nervous, sad, and tense.

Openness to experience (versus closed-mindedness) describes the breadth, depth, originality, and complexity of an individual's mental and experiential life.

Source: As described by John and Srivastava 1999, p. 121.

Rather, these five dimensions represent personality at the broadest level of abstraction, and each dimension summarizes a large number of distinct, more specific personality characteristics" (p. 105).

It is now common practice to refer to each of the Big Five personality traits by a single word. John and Srivastava have offered the description of each of these categories shown in table 7.3. For each factor, an individual respondent can be anywhere on a continuum from fully exhibiting the trait to not exhibiting the trait at all. Thus an individual can exhibit a high degree of conscientiousness by being goal-directed, thinking before acting, and choosing to delay gratification. Alternatively, we can imagine another person who only thinks about the moment without considering longer-term goals or consequences as being low on conscientiousness. Similarly, we can imagine someone who is high on neuroticism as usually being anxious, nervous, sad, and tense, while someone low on this trait would typically seem relaxed and generally happy with the way things are going. Each trait can vary independently from the others, although we will see evidence in later chapters that growing up in a position of severe social disadvantage and stress is often associated with a grouping of certain Big Five traits that in turn are associated with lower educa-tional attainment and as a consequence worse health status over time.

Several authors have developed psychological assessment tools to measure each of these traits within individuals. Costa and McRae (1985) developed the NEO Personality Inventory, which they subsequently refined to include measures of six different aspects of each of the core traits (1995). Gough and Heilbrun (1983) developed what they referred to as the Adjective Check List, a list of approximately 300 adjectives that described individual personality traits. John (1990) used factor analysis to sort a subset of 112 of these adjectives into five groups that corresponded to the Big Five. Based on these analyses, John, Donahue, and Kentle (1991) developed the Big Five Inventory (BFI), a survey instrument consisting of 44 short phrases a subject uses to describe himself or herself, using a five-point response scale from "strongly disagree" to "strongly agree." Sample questions, available online (John 2000), ask subjects to apply this scale to statements such as "I see myself as someone who is ingenious, a deep thinker" or "I see myself as someone who is sometimes shy, inhibited."

When various assessment instruments are compared in assessing personality traits according to the Big Five, they largely provide statistically similar results. Also, when translated into other languages, the same five core traits are consistently identified, suggesting that they do not depend on concepts conveyed only in the English language. The BFI instrument has been translated into nine languages other than English, including Chinese.

In chapter 4 we discussed how the concept of self can differ fundamentally within different cultural contexts. Does this then suggest that the core elements of personality reflected in the Big Five will also vary from culture to culture? Will the expression of traits such as extraversion, conscientiousness, or neuroticism vary based on whether the individual being studied is in an independent culture or an interdependent culture? In their review of how culture and personality intersect, Benet-Martinez and Oishi concluded that "Big Five measures have reliably replicated the same five-factor structure across many different cultures and languages" (2008, p. 546). In a similar review, Triandis and Suh conclude that, "A large body of literature suggests that the Big Five personality factors emerge in various cultures" (2002, p. 133). They caution that there may be traits in addition to the Big Five in other, non-Western cultures that have not yet been identified, as most research has been done in a Western cultural context. They do go on to suggest, however, that "Given that all humans are one species and that personality has genetic roots, the similarities among cultural groups are likely to be greater than the differences" (p. 147).

There is not yet clear evidence establishing a heritable component of the traits measured by the Big Five. Similarly, the traits assessed by it are separate and distinct from one's cognitive ability. McRae and John, early developers of the BFI, state explicitly that "When factored jointly with personality variables, measures of cognitive ability typically form a distinct sixth factor" (1992, p. 191).

Will children exhibit these same traits assessed using the Big Five? If so, how should they be assessed—by asking the children themselves, or by asking the parents or teachers who observe the children on a day-to-day basis? One interesting study by Measelle et al. (2005) used puppets to express certain personality traits to children between the ages of 5 and 7 and then asked the children to indicate the extent to which the trait exhibited by the puppet applied to them. They followed children for up to two years and found substantial consistency over time among a number of the factors measured in this manner.

Most of the research on children, however, has asked parents and teachers to rate the children's traits. Shiner and Caspi (2003) reviewed research in which parents or teachers were asked to assess children's personality using the Big Five traits. They found a high level of consistency in the adults' ability to rate children based on the traits of extraversion, agreeableness, conscientiousness, and neuroticism.

Goldberg (2001) analyzed a data set gathered between 1959 and 1967 in a study of more than 2,500 elementary school children in Hawaii. The original study, done by John Dingman, was an important part of the research effort that resulted in identification of the Big Five traits. In that study, teachers were asked to evaluate children in their class on a series of attributes. Goldberg re-evaluated this data set using only those attributes that later became part of the Big Five assessment.

Working with Goldberg, Hampson et al. (2006) contacted 963 of the individuals in the original study, who now were between 40 and 50 years of age. They gathered data from these adult subjects on a range of health behaviors and health status indicators. They found a significant association between certain of the Big Five traits exhibited as children and health behaviors as adults. For example, children who were rated by their teachers as higher on conscientiousness were less likely to be smokers as adults and more likely to rate their overall health status as better. Similarly, children rated higher on agreeableness were less likely as adults to smoke and less likely to be obese. These findings suggest that personality traits exhibited as children, as perceived by elementary school teachers, are associated with later behaviors as adults that affect health status.

Subsequent analysis of these data by Hampson et al. (2007) determined that many of the effects of childhood personality traits on adult health behaviors were mediated by educational attainment. Subjects rated higher on conscientiousness and agreeableness as elementary school children had a significantly higher level of educational attainment as adults. This higher level of education was, in turn, associated with a healthier behavioral pattern. Thus, childhood personality traits exhibit an effect similar to that of the socioeconomic context in which a child grows up, as discussed in chapter 3.

These results are also strikingly similar to an analysis reported by Friedman et al. (1995). They relied on data compiled in the 1920s by Lewis Terman, an educational psychologist at Stanford University. Terman spent much of his career studying childhood intelligence and developing ways to measure it. He began following more than 1,500 children in California schools, all of whom were rated as intellectually gifted, using what is now called the Stanford-Binet intelligence scale. While Terman's work came several decades before the development of the Big Five scales, one of the specific childhood traits he included in his study of these children was conscientiousness, as rated by the children's teachers and parents. Researchers have been following these subjects on a regular basis since the study was initiated. Friedman found a strong association between conscientiousness as a child and subsequent length of life, with lower rates of smoking explaining part but not all of this difference.

Given the association of personality traits exhibited in childhood with adult health outcomes, one might ask the extent to which these traits remain stable throughout the adult life course. Srivastava et al. (2003) compared two

views on this question: what they referred to as the "biological view" or "plaster hypothesis" that "all personality traits stop changing by age 30" and the "contextualist perspective . . . that changes should be more varied and should persist throughout adulthood" (p. 1041). They used data gathered from an Internet-based survey of 132,515 adults between the ages of 21 and 60 and concluded, "On no Big Five dimension did we find support for the hard plaster hypothesis among both men and women . . . Conscientiousness increased throughout the age range studied, most strongly during the 20s; Agreeableness increased the most during the 30s; and Neuroticism declined with age for women but not much for men. Openness showed small declines with age, and Extraversion declined for women but not men" (p. 1049).

Scales of personality that go beyond the "Big Five"

Not all psychologists or health professionals see the Big Five traits in the same light as the authors we have discussed above. Others have worked to develop scales that they perceive to be of equal reliability from a statistical perspective, but which offer stronger validity in terms of actually predicting outcomes. I will address two of these alternative perspectives: grit and self-efficacy.

Grit: Perseverance and passion for long-term goals

Angela Duckworth is a psychologist at the University of Pennsylvania who has focused her research on two personality traits that she sees as playing a role in predicting one's success in life: grit and self-control. She distinguishes between the two by suggesting that "Grit equips individuals to pursue especially challenging aims over years and even decades. Self-control, in contrast, operates at a more molecular timescale, in the battle against . . . pursuits which bring pleasure in the moment but are immediately regretted" (2014). (She offers some specific examples of these pursuits in the moment: Facebook, Angry Birds, and Krispy Kreme donuts.)

Grit appears to have everything to do with the type of trait assessments Goldberg and John developed. Duckworth's principal criticism of the Big Five approach has to do with its origins in lexical statistics. As Duckworth et al. explain, "A serious limitation of the Big Five taxonomy derives from its roots in the factor analyses of adjectives. Traits for which there are fewer synonyms (or antonyms) tend to be omitted" (2007, p. 1088). They don't question the statistical basis on which the Big Five were developed; rather they suggest that it does not provide a sufficiently inclusive list of important personality traits.

Duckworth et al. define grit as representing "perseverance and passion for long-term goals" (p. 1087). They concur that grit overlaps with conscientiousness as a trait operationalized within the Big Five but suggest that conscientiousness focuses principally on the task or tasks at hand, while grit looks to the long term. John and Srivastava use adjectives such as "efficient," "organized," "thorough," and "deliberate" in delineating conscientiousness (1999, p. 113). While these descriptors certainly seem to be addressing a common theme, as Duckworth suggests they do not describe a trait that persists over time. Grit, on the other hand, describes one's attitude toward the long haul: "individuals high in grit deliberately set for themselves extremely long-term objectives and do not swerve from them—even in the absence of positive feedback" (Duckworth et al. 2007, p. 1089).

Duckworth's research group proposed that grit is strongly associated with high levels of achievement over time in a range of fields, from educational attainment to rigorous military training or a national spelling bee competition. They suggested that, especially when combined with a high level of intelligence, individuals with high levels of grit will apply themselves over the long term, especially in the face of challenges, to attain their goals. The researchers developed and tested a Grit Scale based on subjects' responses to a series of questions and prompts. They found that grit was more strongly associated with the outcomes they measured than either intelligence or any specific Big Five factor.

Self-efficacy

In parallel with the development of the Big Five scales, psychologist Albert Bandura identified a personality trait he referred to as self-efficacy, which "refers to beliefs in one's capabilities to organize and execute the courses of action required to produce given attainments" (1997, p. 3). In his early work on the concept of self-efficacy, Bandura (1977) proposed a series of four processes through which individuals develop their own sense of efficacy in identifying and attaining goals.

A principal means through which one begins to perceive a sense of efficacy is what Bandura refers to as performance accomplishment. As a child develops her or his cognitive capacities, she or he will begin to see a pattern linking behavior and outcome. Over time, the child learns that a certain behavior can be expected to result in a specific outcome. Sometimes the outcome is perceived as positive and sometimes as negative. The key is the causal connection the child makes between the behavior and the outcome, allowing the child to internalize an expectation of her or his own capacity to accomplish certain outcomes in the future. Over time, the stronger the sense of efficacy an individual develops, the more challenging the outcome she or he is willing to try for, the greater the effort she or he will expend, and the greater the persistence she or he will invest in attaining the outcome.

Of course, not all individuals experience a pattern of success in their efforts as they grow: For a variety of reasons, often having more to do with the environment in which one is growing up than with one's innate physical or intellectual strengths, a pattern of failure to attain the intended outcome may pervade over a pattern of success. These individuals are prone to develop a substantially lower sense of self-efficacy and accordingly are likely to be less willing to take on challenging goals and prone to giving up sooner in the face of challenges.

A second mechanism through which individuals develop this sense of their own efficacy is what Bandura refers to as vicarious experience: "Seeing others perform threatening activities without adverse consequences can generate expectations in observers that they too will improve if they intensify and persist in their efforts" (1977, p. 197). In a sense, an individual comes to model his or her own behavior on observations of others trying and succeeding with challenging tasks (or conversely, trying and failing): "If he (or she) can do it, so can I. I'm as good as him (or her)." Sometimes the person taken on as a model is a peer to whom one feels equivalent. Other times the model may be a mentor or role model.

A third mechanism for enhancing self-efficacy is through verbal persuasion by others—most typically a parent, teacher, or mentor. Repeated messages of "You can do it if you just try hard enough," when heard from someone one respects and whose opinion one values, can strengthen one's previously internalized sense of capacity and efficacy. How the encouragement is phrased can influence how effective the encouragement is in persuading the listener. This finding is consistent with the work of Dweck and others described in chapter 6.

The fourth mechanism identified by Bandura is emotional arousal. Strong emotional arousal will often trigger a response in the amygdala, which can then affect cognitive processes. If that arousal is based on anxiety or fear of failure, perceived efficacy at attaining an outcome may be diminished. On the other hand if the response involves more positive emotions such as excitement or positive anticipation, perceived efficacy may be enhanced.

Bandura points out that, of these four mechanisms, performance accomplishment, which he later refers to as "enactive mastery experience" (1997, p. 80), has the strongest impact. While the other mechanisms may enhance perceived self-efficacy, if the principal pattern of experience has been one of failure, the others may not be able to overcome that perception.

The issue of self-efficacy, and the means for others to influence one's perceived level of efficacy, is especially important in the educational experience. In a focused discussion of the role of self-efficacy in the educational context, Bandura describes how "Students' beliefs in their efficacy to regulate their own learning and to master academic activities determine their aspirations, level of motivation, and academic accomplishments" (1993, p. 117).

In the school environment, both self-efficacy and actual cognitive abilities will affect how well a student does. Students from a disadvantaged socioeconomic background can enter school with reduced cognitive abilities when compared with more advantaged students of the same age. If they were also to enter school with a reduced sense of self-efficacy, they would be at especially high risk of reinforcing those negative perceptions. When faced with the challenges of learning new material in school, "people who harbor self-doubts about their capabilities slacken their efforts or give up quickly. Those who have a strong belief in their capabilities exert greater effort when they fail to master the challenge" (p. 131). If a child were also to view peers succeeding where he or she has failed and then to begin to sense negative rather than positive expectations from the teacher, the adverse impact on perceived efficacy can be magnified.

Bandura goes on to underscore the importance of this process in the educational experience. "By the choices they make, people cultivate different competencies, interests, and social networks that determine life courses. Any factor that influences choice behavior can profoundly affect the direction of personal development" (p. 135).

Bandura went on to research the potential social impacts on children in school of impaired self-efficacy coupled with academic weakness. He found that

> children who have a high sense of academic and self-regulatory efficacy behave more prosocially, are more popular, and experience less rejection by their peers than do children who believe they lack these forms of academic efficacy . . . The impact of children's disbelief in their academic efficacy on socially discordant behavior becomes stronger as they grow older . . . Students who doubt their social as well as their intellectual efficacy are likely to gravitate to peers who do not subscribe to academic values and lifestyles. Over time, growing self-doubts in cognitive competencies foreclose many occupational life courses. (p. 138)

Mental illness and disorders of personality

For much of the last century, many of those who have engaged in the study of personality have focused on how to describe and classify disorders of personality. Recall that both Sigmund Freud and Erik Erikson were psychotherapists who developed their "stages of development" in order to describe what they considered to be the normal process of psychological development. Based on these normal developmental processes they then described the forms of mental illness that often resulted from disruptions to these processes. One thing they had in common was the view that mental illness is often a consequence of early developmental abnormalities.

Mental illness has been recognized for centuries. Shakespeare seemed to have a special interest in it, giving characters such as King Lear and Macbeth behaviors that would today be classified as mental illness. For much of the 19th century, mental illness as seen in Western societies was divided into two broad categories: psychosis and neurosis. As described by the *Oxford English Dictionary*, psychosis was viewed as "severe mental illness, characterized by loss of contact with reality (in the form of delusions and hallucinations)." By contrast, the *OED* defines neurosis as a "psychological disorder in which there is disabling or distressing anxiety, without severe disorganization or distortion of behaviour or personality."

We no longer see these terms used in categorizing mental illness. Beginning in the mid-20th century, the organization that was to become the American Psychiatric Association began collaborating with the US government to develop a systematic nomenclature of mental illness. This effort was expanded following World War II and resulted in 1952 in the publication of the first edition of the *Diagnostic and Statistical Manual: Mental Disorders*, referred to as *DSM-I*. In the decades since then, the *DSM* has undergone a series of revisions, with *DSM-5* being published in 2013. In this updated edition, previous divisions of mental illnesses into distinct groups, referred to as Axes, was discontinued, and different types of mental illnesses were listed with descriptors of the variations that might exist within a specific illness. Some of the principal illnesses identified in *DSM-5*, with specific examples given for some illnesses, are shown in table 7.4.

Looking at the disorders listed in the table, and considering the common views of the origins of mental illness as described by Freud and Erikson, two questions seem central to our understanding.

1) To what extent are these disorders caused by disruptive social or interpersonal experiences, especially during childhood and early development?
2) To what extent are these disorders caused by inherited genetic abnormalities?

TABLE 7.4. Categories of Mental Illnesses Described in *DSM-5,* with Examples of Specific Illnesses within a Category

Neurodevelopmental Disorders
 Global Developmental Delay
 Autism Spectrum Disorder
 Attention-Deficit/Hyperactivity Disorder

Schizophrenia Spectrum and Other Psychotic Disorders

Bipolar and Related Disorders

Depressive Disorders

Anxiety Disorders
 Social Anxiety Disorder (Social Phobia)
 Panic Disorder
 Agoraphobia
 Generalized Anxiety Disorder

Obsessive-Compulsive and Related Disorders

Trauma- and Stressor-Related Disorders
 Post-Traumatic Stress Disorder
 Acute Stress Disorder
 Adjustment Disorders

Neurocognitive Disorders
 Parkinson's Disease
 Huntington's Disease

Personality Disorders
 General Personality Disorder
 Paranoid Personality Disorder
 Antisocial Personality Disorder
 Borderline Personality Disorder
 Narcissistic Personality Disorder
 Dependent Personality Disorder

Source: American Psychiatric Association 2013.

Some of these disorders have a clear genetic origin. For example, among the neurocognitive disorders listed, both Huntington's disease and certain forms of Parkinson's disease have recognized genetic abnormalities as their cause. These genetic mutations can be passed on to one's children, who are then likely to develop the disease. By contrast, posttraumatic stress disorder and acute stress disorder are responses to extremely stressful life experiences, with no associated genetic abnormality.

Scientists as well have psychotherapists have been discussing the causal role of genetics vs. life experiences for many of the other diseases. For some, there appears to be a strong consensus that inherited genetic abnormalities play a central role in disease causation. This is true for diseases such as schizophrenia, bipolar disorders, and some depressive disorders. A consortium of researchers recently identified a series of genetic mutations that appear to be involved in several of these illnesses (Cross-Disorder Group 2013). Analyzing the pattern of single nucleotide polymorphisms among about 33,000 adults with mental illness and 28,000 adults without known illness, all of European ancestry, they noted significant overlap in the genetic abnormalities associated with bipolar disorder, major depressive disorder, and schizophrenia, leading the authors to conclude that "Accumulating evidence, including that from clinical, epidemiological, and molecular genetic studies, suggests that some genetic risk factors are shared between neuropsychiatric disorders" (p. 1377).

In contrast to those disorders with a defined genetic causation, there is also broad agreement that certain disruptions in early child development can lead to symptoms of mental illness that may last well into adulthood. Going beyond Freud's concepts of psychosexual aspects of child development, psychologists John Bowlby and Mary Ainsworth developed a theory, referred to as attachment theory, that identifies a child's healthy attachment to his or her mother during infancy as central to developing a healthy personality (Bretherton 1992). As described by Bowlby, "attachment behaviour is conceived as a class of behaviour distinct from feeding behaviour and sexual behaviour and of at least an equal significance in human life" (1977, p. 204). Bowlby goes on to explain, "The key point of my thesis is that there is a strong causal relationship between an individual's experiences with his parents and his later capacity to make affectional bonds, and that certain common variations in that capacity, manifesting themselves in marital problems and trouble with children as well as in neurotic symptoms and personality disorders, can be attributed to common variations in the way parents perform their parental roles" (p. 206).

Bowbly incorporated into his theory much of the research of Mary Ainsworth (Ainsworth and Bowlby 1991). Ainsworth studied the relationship between infants and their mothers, both in Africa and in Baltimore, Maryland. Through careful observation of the interactions over time between mother and infant, she identified clear patterns of sensitive and supportive parenting as well as patterns of anxious and disconnected parenting. The child's subsequent responses to these different caring patterns during the first months and years of life resulted in differing patterns of behavior toward the parent and toward others. These abnormal childhood responses, they hypothesized, would come to be associated with potentially serious disorders of personality and interpersonal relationships as adults. Responding to critics who took more of a traditional Freudian view of the childhood origins of mental illness, Bowlby commented,

> Throughout this century debate has raged about the role of childhood experiences in the causation of psychiatric disturbance. Not only have traditionally minded psychiatrists been skeptical of their relevance but psychoanalysts have been at sixes and sevens about them . . . No one engaged in child psychiatry, better termed family psychiatry, can possible share such a view. In a great majority of cases not only is there evidence of disturbed family relationships but the emotional problems of the parents, derived from their own unhappy childhoods, commonly loom large. (p. 205)

This perspective voiced by Bowlby will be of particular significance when we discuss in chapter 10 the long-term impact of adverse childhood experiences.

Summary

We began this chapter by comparing different historical perspectives on the process by which personality develops, from birth through either adolescence (as seen by Freud) or throughout the life course (as seen by Erikson). We then described various ways psychologists have proposed conceptualizing and categorizing personality according to specific traits. There is no single best way to connect the developmental process with the traits exhibited in adolescence and adulthood. Nor is there a single best way to define and measure the different types of traits people exhibit. A constant factor across these various theories, though, is the importance personality has for affecting both behavior and well-being. Similarly, many of the theorists, principal among them Freud, Erikson, and Bandura, also proposed that we gain a better understanding of how mental health or educational professionals can work with individuals who exhibit mental illness or negative personality traits by identifying both the roots of those traits and the steps one can take to overcome them. While a number of these illnesses have distinct genetic causes, it remains key in this therapeutic process for the person offering this support to enable a feeling of trust and respect in the person receiving that support and a belief that, through consistent, hard work, past barriers can be overcome and newly adopted goals realized.

REFERENCES

Ainsworth, M. S., & Bowlby, J. 1991. An ethological approach to personality development. American Psychologist 46(4): 333–41.

Allport, G. W., & Odbert, H. S. 1936. Trait names: A psycho-lexical study. Psychological Monographs 47(211).

American Psychiatric Association. 2013. Diagnostic and Statistical Manual of Mental Disorders. 5th edition. Arlington, VA: American Psychiatric Association.

American Psychological Association. Glossary of psychological terms. Available at www.apa.org /research/action/glossary.aspx, accessed 5/26/14.

Bandura, A. 1977. Self-efficacy: Toward a unifying theory of behavioral change. Psychological Review 84(2): 191-215.

———. 1993. Perceived self-efficacy in cognitive development and functioning. Educational Psychologist 28(2): 117-48.

———. 1997. Self-Efficacy: The Exercise of Control. New York: W.H. Freeman and Company.

Benet-Martínez, V., & Oishi, S. 2008. Culture and personality. In John, O. P., Robins, R.W., & Pervin, L. A., eds. Handbook of Personality: Theory and Research. New York: Guildford Press.

Bowlby, J. 1977. The making and breaking of affectional bonds. I. Aetiology and psychopathology in the light of attachment theory. British Journal of Psychiatry 130(3): 201-10.

Bretherton, I. 1992. The origins of Attachment Theory: John Bowlby and Mary Ainsworth. Developmental Psychology 28(5): 759-75.

Cattell, R. B., Eber H. W., & Tatsuoka, M. M. 1970. Handbook for the Sixteen Personality Factor Questionnaire. Champaign, IL: IPAT.

Costa, P. T., & McCrae, R. R. 1985. The NEO Personality Inventory Manual. Odessa, FL: Psychological Assessment Resources.

———. 1995. Domains and facets: Hierarchical personality assessment using the Revised NEO Personality Inventory. Journal of Personality Assessment 64(1): 21-50.

Cross-Disorder Group of the Psychiatric Genomics Consortium. 2013. Identification of risk loci with shared effects on five major psychiatric disorders: A genome-wide analysis. The Lancet 381 (9875): 1371-79.

Duckworth, A. Research statement: The Duckworth Lab, available at https://sites.sas.upenn.edu/duckworth/pages/research, accessed 6/11/14.

Duckworth, A. L., Peterson, C., Matthews, M. D., & Kelly, D. R. 2007.Grit: Perseverance and passion for long-term goals. Journal of Personality and Social Psychology 92(6): 1087-1101.

Erikson, E. H. 1963. Childhood and Society. 2nd edition. New York: W.W. Norton & Company.

Erikson, E. H., & Erikson, J. M. 1997. The Life Cycle Completed: Extended Version with New Chapters on the Ninth Stage of Development. New York: W. W. Norton

Fleming, J. S. 2004a. Erikson's psychosocial developmental stages. In Psychological Perspectives on Human Development, available at http://swppr.org/Textbook/Contents.html, accessed 5/31/14.

———. 2004b. Freud and the psychodynamic approach to development. In Psychological Perspectives on

Human Development, available at http://swppr.org/Textbook/Contents.html, accessed 5/31/14.

Freud, S. 1975[1905]. Three Essays on the Theory of Sexuality. Translated by James Strachey. New York: Basic Books.

Friedman, H. S., Tucker, J. S., Schwartz, J. E., et al. 1995. Childhood conscientiousness and longevity: Health behaviors and cause of death. Journal of Personality and Social Psychology 68(4): 696-703.

Gilligan, C. 1993. In a Different Voice: Psychological Theory and Women's Development. Reissued edition of 1982 edition. Cambridge, MA: Harvard University Press.

Goldberg, L. R. 1990. An alternative "Description of Personality": The Big-Five factor structure. Journal of Personality and Social Psychology 59(6): 1216-29.

———. 2001. Analyses of Digman's child-personality data: Derivation of Big-Five factor scores from each of six samples. Journal of Personality 69(5): 709-43.

Gough, H. G., & Heilbrun, A. B. Jr. 1983. The Adjective Checklist Manual. Palo Alto, CA: Consulting Psychologists Press.

Hampson, S. E., Goldberg, L. R., Vogt, T. M., & Dubanoski, J. P. 2006. Forty years on: Teachers' assessments of children's personality traits predict self-reported health behaviors and outcomes at midlife. Health Psychology 25(1): 57-64.

———. 2007. Mechanisms by which childhood personality traits influence adult health status: Educational attainment and healthy behaviors. Health Psychology 26(1): 121-5.

John, O. P. 1990. The "Big Five" factor taxonomy: Dimensions of personality in the natural language and in questionnaires. In Pervin, L. A., ed. Handbook of Personality: Theory and Research, 66-100. New York: Guilford Press.

———. 2000. The Big Five Personality Test, available at www.outofservice.com/bigfive/, accessed 6/7/14.

John, O. P., Donahue, E. M., & Kentle, R. L. 1991. The Big Five Inventory: Versions 4a and 54. Berkeley, CA: Institute of Personality and Social Research.

John, O. P., & Srivastava, S. 1999. The Big Five trait taxonomy: History, measurement, and theoretical perspectives. In Pervin, L. A., & Johns, O. P., eds. Handbook of Personality: Theory and Research, 2nd ed., pp. 102-38. New York: Guilford Press.

McCrae, R. R., & John, O. P. 1992. An introduction to the five-factor model and its applications. Journal of Personality 60(2): 175-215.

Measelle, J. R., John, O. P., Ablow, J. C., Cowan, P. A., & Cowan, C. P. 2005. Can children provide coherent, stable, and valid self-reports on the Big Five dimensions? A longitudinal study from ages 5 to 7. Journal of Personality and Social Psychology 89(1): 90-106.

Norman, W. T. 1967. 2,800 personality trait descriptors: Normative operating characteristics for a university population. Ann Arbor, MI: Department of Psychology, University of Michigan.

Oxford English Dictionary online, available at www.oed.com, accessed 5/30/14.

Shiner, R. L., & Caspi, A. 2003. Personality differences in childhood and adolescence: Measurement,

development, and consequences. Journal of Child Psychology and Psychiatry 44: 2-31.

Srivastava, S., John, O. P, Gosling, S. D., & Potter, J. 2003. Development of personality in early and middle adulthood: Set like plaster or persistent change? Journal of Personality and Social Psychology 84(5): 1041-53.

Tough, P. 2012. How Children Succeed: Grit, Curiosity, and the Hidden Power of Character. Boston, MA: Houghton Mifflin Harcourt.

Triandis, H. C., & Suh, E. M. 2002. Cultural influence on personality. Annual Review of Psychology 53: 133-60.

CHAPTER 8

The Brain and Behavior

Behavior involves an individual's response to a perceived stimulus. There are three core steps in the process of behavior: perception of the stimulus, interpretation of that stimulus, and response to that interpretation. This pattern is involved in a wide range of behaviors, from newborn infants sucking a pacifier more slowly when they heard sounds that were in the language of their mother to adults with lower levels of education deciding more often to light up a cigarette.

While the association between adult educational attainment and smoking involves issues of motivation and personality, the newborn responding to the sound of the mother's language has not yet developed these characteristics. For both the adult smoker and the newborn infant sucking on the pacifier, however, each of the steps in the process of these behaviors, from perception to response, involves the body's nervous system.

The perception of stimuli usually relies on the various sensory organs and their neural connections to the brain. The interpretation of the sensory impulses received by the brain involves other parts of the brain involved in memory and meaning. Finally, any action, from blinking one's eyes or making a sound with one's mouth to moving one's hand and arm to catch a baseball or opening a book to study for an exam, involves neural impulses generated in the brain's motor cortex or other parts of the brain involved in muscular stimulation.

Accordingly, the first step in understanding the roots of human behavior is gaining an understanding of the development as well as the structure and function of the brain and nervous system. To introduce this concept, consider the processes involved when we go to an Internet site to obtain information or carry out a transaction.

The importance of communication between information sources: On the Internet and in the human brain

For better or worse, the Internet has become an increasingly prevalent part of our lives, in a range of capacities and contexts. We have come to expect a website to be readily available (assuming we have the means of accessing it) and to respond quickly and accurately to our inquiries and requests. Sometimes, though, we encounter a site that is slow in responding or that gives us an error message, indicating (much to our frustration) that it cannot proceed with the transaction.

One of the most publicized of these website failures occurred in October 2013, when the federal government opened Healthcare.gov as a means of creating a new health insurance marketplace for individuals and families to acquire health insurance under the guidelines and rules of the Affordable Care Act. Unfortunately, things did not go smoothly at first. No sooner had the website opened for business than reports started rolling in about how poorly it functioned. Users had trouble getting onto the website, and those who tried to create accounts were often left in limbo. It often took an extraordinarily long time for a window to load,

and users often obtained incomplete or inaccurate information. Even after many of these problems were fixed, there continued to be problems for participating insurance companies in getting accurate data about those who had enrolled in their plans, and the new enrollees often had trouble getting verification of coverage from the insurer.

Looking at these problems from the perspective of the user, Healthcare.gov simply didn't work. This perspective is illustrated in figure 8.1.

From the point of view of the outside user trying to get Healthcare.gov to respond, the problem was simple: The website was malfunctioning. A common perception in news reports approached the new website as a single entity with a single function—making health insurance available to the potential purchaser.

Subsequent news stories, federal reports, and policy analyses demonstrated that this view, of a single website that simply didn't work, was not fully accurate. A more accurate understanding of the many and complex factors that went into Healthcare.gov is shown in figure 8.2.

Healthcare.gov was actually both a computer server that interacted electronically with a user on the web and a portal for the transfer of information among a wide host of other servers and data files. When an individual applied for coverage, the federal Center for Medicare and Medicaid Services automatically communicated with a range of federal, state, and private agencies to verify eligibility for coverage. As described on the informational website provided by CMS, when you logged on to Healthcare.gov:

- Social Security may verify your Social Security numbers and citizenship status.
- The US Department of Homeland Security may verify your immigration status.
- The Internal Revenue Service may verify your household income and family size; the income of household members may also be verified with the Social Security Adminis-

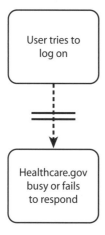

FIGURE 8.1. Healthcare.gov: From the Perspective of the User

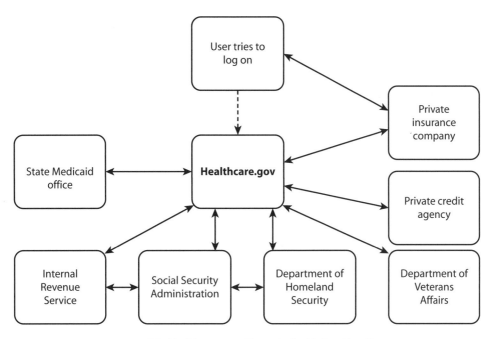

FIGURE 8.2. Healthcare.gov: From the Inside Looking Out

tration and with a consumer credit reporting agency.

- A consumer credit reporting agency may verify your employment information.
- The employers listed on your application may verify your eligibility for employer-sponsored health plans.
- The State Medical Assistance (Medicaid) office, the Children's Health Insurance Program (CHIP), the US Department of Veterans Affairs, Medicare, Peace Corps, US Department of Defense (for TRICARE), US Department of Health and Human Services, the Office of Personnel Management, and the Small Business Health Option Programs that operate in your state may verify your eligibility for and/or enrollment in health coverage programs.

Each of these agencies or organizations had its own computer server, with its own web address and its own security and communication protocols. As figure 8.2 illustrates, assuring the proper functioning of the complex web of com-munications among the various servers was equally important as the proper functioning of the servers themselves. Healthcare.gov was a complex network of central information sources and interconnecting webs of communication, and it was largely these interagency communications that malfunctioned, not the computer servers themselves. For example, in re-evaluating the expected enrollment in private health insurance and in Medicaid under the Affordable Care Act, the Congressional Budget Office (2014, p. 114) described how "the exchanges operated by the federal government have struggled to transfer application information to state agencies for people who might be eligible for Medicaid or CHIP." It was the neural connections between the servers that malfunctioned much more so than the servers themselves.

The human brain can be seen as analogous to this structural arrangement. From one perspective, looking at the brain as a single functional unit, we might see what is shown in figure 8.3.

To look at the brain, however, as a single functional unit would be analogous to looking

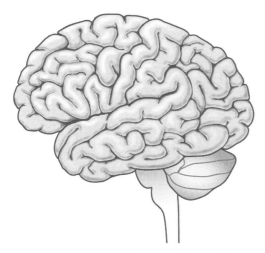

**Outer surface of
left side of brain**

FIGURE 8.3. The Human Brain

at the webpage of Healthcare.gov as a single computer server. Just as Healthcare.gov has multiple functional units with complex interconnections among them, so the human brain has a wide range of functional units spread through the tissue of the organ itself as well as an incredibly complex web of communications links. In addition to these multiple units, the brain is structured and functions at multiple levels. In much the same way that a computer server will have both program algorithms that govern how data input is managed and backup files to store old data in case one ever needs to retrieve them, the brain has conscious and unconscious control mechanisms that maintain overall functional control as well as substantial memory capacity for the storage and retrieval of old information.

The principal functional units in the brain are referred to as the cortices (with one unit called a cortex). Each of the human body's five core senses (taste, smell, touch, vision, and hearing) has a cortical area that receives the sensory impulses coming from the body. Taste, based on the stimulation of receptors in the mouth and tongue, travels over a series of nerves that connect the mouth to the gustatory cortex of the brain, located within the frontal lobe. Sensations of smell travel over the olfactory nerve from the nasal cavities to the olfactory cortex, part of the temporal lobe. The area of the brain that handles sensory input from the eyes is the visual cortex; the section that handles sound is the auditory cortex; and the area that receives tactile stimuli from the nerves at the periphery of the body is the sensory cortex. The part of the brain that sends instructions to the muscles regarding movement is the motor cortex. These areas are illustrated in figure 8.5 below. There are also areas whose principal function is thought and reasoning. These include the association cortex and the prefrontal cortex.

There are also localized parts of the brain that function at more of an unconscious level. The hippocampus plays a major role in memory storage and retrieval, the amygdala plays a central role in feeling and responding to emotion, the thalamus controls consciousness and sleep, and the hypothalamus monitors and controls physiologic functions such as body temperature and response to stress.

While each of these sections of the brain tissue has an important function in itself, the brain cannot function adequately if the various sections fail to communicate with each other quickly and efficiently. This communication requires a web of nerve fibers called axons. These axonal connections allow us to perform the many and complex tasks involved with human existence. To illustrate, let us consider two core functions of the human brain: understanding spoken language and reading. The activities involved in these two functions are illustrated in figure 8.4.

First let us consider hearing spoken language. The ears sense sound waves and send information about that sensory input over specialized nerve pathways to the auditory cortex, an area of the brain that has developed the specialized capacity to receive this input. As part of the process of learning to recognize language,

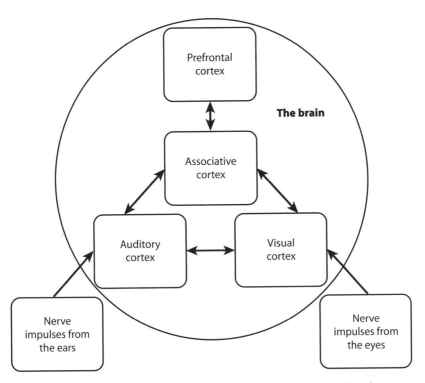

FIGURE 8.4. How the Human Brain Handles Spoken Language and Reading

infants start to be able to distinguish certain sound patterns as representing words, as distinct from those patterns that simply represent noise. This process actually begins in the womb as the developing fetus hears the sound of the mother speaking. As described in chapter 1, Moon et al. (2013) tested whether newborn infants could distinguish vowel sounds from the language spoken by their mother from vowel sounds spoken in a different language. Based on different rates of sucking on a pacifier in response to the sounds, they found clear evidence that infants have already developed the basics of sound recognition by the time they are born.

In order to develop language, an infant must learn to associate a certain sound or groups of sounds with a visual image of an object. For example, to understand the word *dog*, an infant must recognize this unique sound when it is spoken and associate it with the four-legged animal it represents. Fernald et al. (2013) studied

the development of language perception in 18–24 month old infants by playing the sound of a spoken word for the infant to hear and immediately displaying two pictures: one an image of the object associated with the word and another that was unrelated to the word. They were able to watch the direction of the infant's gaze after hearing the word, to see if it was directed to the picture of the object associated with it. They used words such as *baby, doggy, birdie,* and *ball.* They found that these infants were able quickly to recognize many of the words, but that children from families of lower socioeconomic status (SES) recognized fewer words on average than children from higher-SES families—something that will take on added importance when we consider below the neural systems and connections involved in learning to read.

Figure 8.5 illustrates the parts of the human brain involved in language. It shows the visual

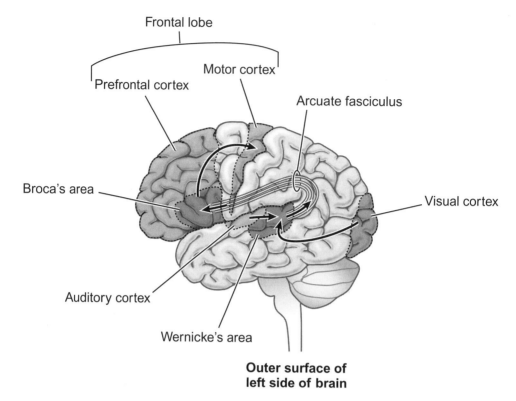

FIGURE 8.5. The Parts of the Brain Involved in Language

cortex at the back of the brain, the auditory cortex on the side of the brain, and an area that associates visual and auditory stimuli, here labeled Wernicke's area. As an infant repeatedly hears a word and sees the object the word is intended to represent, the auditory stimulus is coupled with the visual stimulus in Wernicke's area, and that association is then stored in memory. At a later time the infant can hear the word without also seeing the image and, through the connection between the auditory cortex and Wernicke's area, retrieve from memory the image of the object the word represents.

Beyond simply recognizing a word, an infant must also give meaning to the word. For example, an infant might associate the word *dog* or *doggy* with experiences it has had with dogs, whether real dogs or imaginary dogs seen on the pages of a book. The infant's brain does this by connecting the associative memory created in Wernicke's area with another area located in the frontal lobe, referred to as Broca's area. The frontal cortex of the brain is responsible for intellectual processes as well as the initiation of motor activity. The area referred to as the prefrontal cortex manages intellectual activity such as abstract reasoning and planning future activity. Broca's area is part of the prefrontal cortex.

A next step in language development is for the infant to be able to speak the words it has learned. Speaking involves the creation of nerve impulses in the motor cortex of the brain, which is also part of the frontal cortex, and the transmission of these impulses to the complex system of muscles in the mouth, vocal cords, and lungs that allows us to form spoken words. Thus learning both to understand language spoken by others and then to speak the language oneself involves a complex series of communications among the various cortical areas involved, as illustrated in figure 8.4 above. As was the case with Healthcare.gov, the proper functioning of these activities depends at least as much on efficient communication among the various cortical areas as it does on having those local cortical areas function properly.

The final process we will address as part of this discussion is learning to read, a process that typically takes place after infancy, in early childhood. A necessary precursor to learning to read a language is first learning to hear and speak that language. A child who has never learned the sound and associated meaning of the word *book* can look at the printed letters *b-o-o-k* and yet derive no meaning from that visual image. A child who has previously learned to hear and to speak the word, upon seeing the printed letters in sequence, can quickly recognize the meaning associated with that visual image. The child's brain does this through a rapid sequence of communication between the visual cortex, the associative area of Wernicke's area, and Broca's area, where the meaning associated with the word is stored. If all these communications go smoothly, the child understands the meaning of the word and how it relates to the words coming before and after it. As part of this process of comprehension, the brain sends signals to the muscles controlling the movement of the eyes to scan the printed words that follow.

Once again, in order to read quickly, these communication paths among the various cortical areas involved must work efficiently. Scientists studying the function of the brain have identified specialized nerve fibers involved in the communications processes involved in language and reading. The arcuate fasciculus is one of these communications links. It is a large bundle of nerve fibers that connects Wernicke's area to Broca's area as one of the principal communications circuits involved in language and reading. To fully understand the dual importance of the cortical areas of the brain and the communications circuits such as the arcuate

fasciculus that link them together, let us consider how these different functional parts of the brain develop embryonically.

The development of the human brain, from embryo to organ

From the fertilization of a female ovum by a male sperm, a process of rapid cellular division and differentiation is triggered that will eventually result in the complete, complex organism we know as the human infant. Within a short period of time after the development of the embryo, the various organ systems begin to differentiate. One of the most important of these is the nervous system, which begins to develop a tubular structure known as the neural tube. Within the developing neural tube, some embryonic stem cells (those cells with the potential to become any of a range of precursor cells, which in turn differentiate into the various organ systems) become neural stem cells. These cells will then undergo further differentiation into two broad categories of precursor cells: neuroblasts, which will become neurons within the nervous system, and glial precursor cells, which will develop into the various types of cell that support the function of neurons without actually being involved in the process of transmitting neural impulses.

As the neuroblasts that will form the brain undergo further differentiation, they begin a process of migration to specific locations within the developing brain. This migration process is triggered by a combination of chemical messages being released in the different brain centers and portions of the neuroblast that sense the presence of these chemical signals. Groups of neuroblasts clump together and will eventually become the various functional areas of the brain such as those we have described that are involved in language and reading.

Once the neuroblasts have migrated to their functional area, the next stage in the process is the development of connections, both among the specialized cells in the same area and with specialized cells in other areas. The cells develop these connections by sending out narrow projections of the cell, with a specialized receptor called the growth cone at the leading edge of the projection. The growth cone senses chemical signals coming from other, more distant cells and continues to grow in an elongated projection in the direction of those chemical signals. As described by Duboc on the website "The Brain From Top to Bottom," "Probably one of the most amazing things about the way the nervous system develops is how the growing axons find their target cells, even though these cells are often located millimetres or even centimetres away (a vast distance on this scale). The source of this ability is the growth cone, a structure at the tip of each elongating axon."

The axon is the elongated portion of the neuron that connects it with more distant cells. In addition to this connection, the cell also develops numerous connections with similar cells in the same functional area. These connections are made through numerous, branching, shorter connections called dendrites. Thus a neuron may have an axon, connecting it to more distant cells, and multiple dendrites, connecting it to adjacent cells with a similar function. These structures, and the steps leading to their differentiation, are illustrated in figure 8.6.

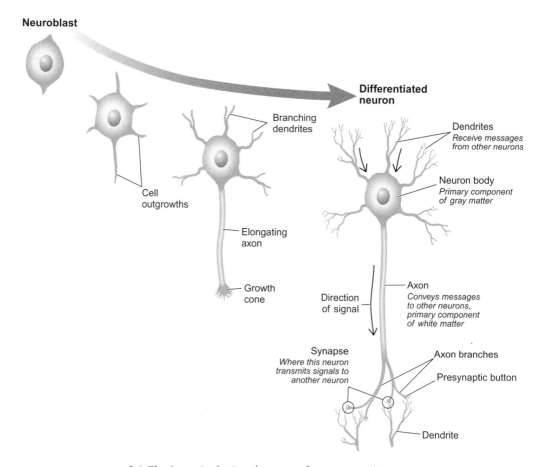

FIGURE 8.6. The Stages in the Development of a Neuron in the Human Brain

In the fully differentiated neuron, the web of dendrites extending from the cell connects it to similar neurons in the immediate vicinity, while the axon can extend great distances (in relative terms) to link the cell to other functional centers of neurons. The grouping of similar neurons in an area of the brain creates a functional unit, while the collective neurons create the pathways for this functional center to communicate with other functional centers. In the case of language and reading described above, the visual cortex, auditory cortex, Wernicke's area, and Broca's area each represents a local functional unit, while the arcuate fasciculus that connects Wernicke's area to Broca's area is an example of an essential communication pathway. This developmental process, with clumps of neurons linking together through their dendrites while also communicating with more distant centers, is illustrated in figure 8.7.

We see in the first panel the differentiation and subsequent proliferation of two separate groups of neurons. As they grow and mature, the cells on the left develop extensive webs of dendrites so as to link together as well as a series of axons that, in response to chemical signals being given off by the cells on the right, elongate in the direction of these cells until they actually make contact with them. As the area on the left begins to carry out its specialized function, the frequency of its axonal communications with the area on the right increases.

One of the most interesting things about the structure and function of these types of axonal connections is that, the more often they convey messages over their length to the associated areas, the better they get at conveying these messages. The more an axon is used to communicate, the faster those communications become, with increased efficiency of communication between the functional areas. I address this aspect of axonal communication below as part the discussion of axonal myelination.

These processes, initiated as part of embryonic development and carried out through fetal development, lead to the development of the human brain as a complex system of specialized cortical areas connected by extensive communication webs. It is typical to refer to the various local aggregation of neurons that comprise the cortical areas as gray matter and the branching groups of axons that connect the various cortical areas as white matter. When examining the brain in cross section using MRI or other types of imaging, the cortical areas appear as gray, while the axons connecting them appear as white. These appearances are shown in figure 8.8.

One of the fascinating things about the way the human brain has developed from an evolutionary perspective is how the development of our brains differs from that of other primates that have not developed the same level of language, communication, and intellectual capacity. Buckner and Krienen (2013) have described the evolution of the brain structure of placental mammals from an original common ancestor. They examine the relative position of three essential sensory areas of the brain: the visual cortex, the auditory cortex, and the somatosensory cortex (the area that receives sensory input from the nerves in the periphery of the body that sense stimuli such as touch and pressure). They compare the positioning of these cortical regions in a range of modern-day mammals, from mice and hedgehogs through the great apes and humans, and conclude that the relative positioning of these areas in the brain has remained fairly constant throughout evolutionary history. As with humans and other primates, the visual cortex of hedgehogs and mice is at the posterior of the brain, the auditory cortex is at the midlateral aspect of the brain, and the somatosensory area is in the upper-mid portion of the brain.

While the positioning of these and other cortical areas has not changed throughout evolution, what has changed dramatically is the overall size of the brain. As described by Buckner

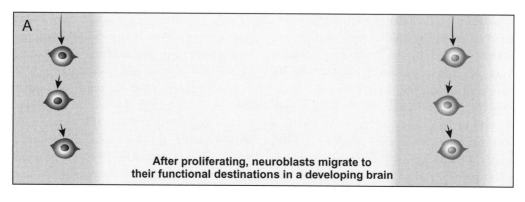

A

After proliferating, neuroblasts migrate to
their functional destinations in a developing brain

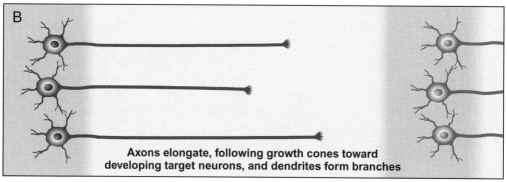

B

Axons elongate, following growth cones toward
developing target neurons, and dendrites form branches

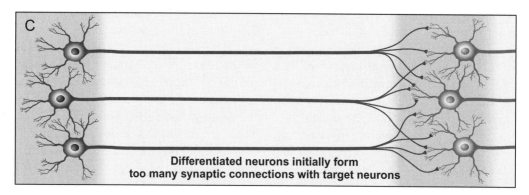

C

Differentiated neurons initially form
too many synaptic connections with target neurons

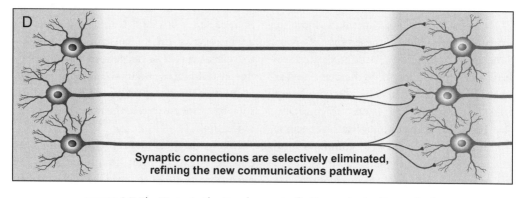

D

Synaptic connections are selectively eliminated,
refining the new communications pathway

FIGURE 8.7. The Stages in the Development of a Neuron in the Human Brain

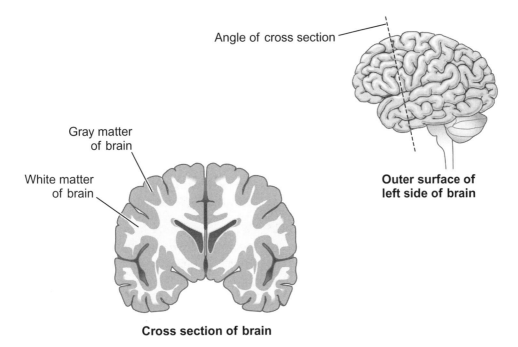

Angle of cross section

Gray matter
of brain

White matter
of brain

**Outer surface of
left side of brain**

Cross section of brain

FIGURE 8.8. Cross Section of the Human Brain, showing Gray Matter and White Matter

and Krienen, the human brain is more than three times larger than the brain of the chimpanzee. Despite this difference in overall size, the absolute size of the principal sensory cortices is almost the same in humans and chimpanzees. It may well be that the chimpanzee is able to sense visual and auditory stimuli just as well as humans. What makes us a fundamentally different species is what our brains do with this sensory input.

If our brains are three times larger than that of the chimpanzee and yet our sensory cortices are about the same size, what makes up the rest of the extra brain area that humans have but chimpanzees don't? Buckner and Krienen conclude that it is the vast web of communication between cortical areas, which they refer to as the "association cortex," that differentiates the human brain from that of the chimpanzee.

The expanded association cortex contains networks operating in parallel with the canonical sensory-motor [cortices] in the service of information processing that is detached from sensory perception and motor actions—what one might term 'internal mentation'. This is an intriguing possibility because it brings to the forefront the kinds of information processing that humans do so well such as remembering, imagining the future, social judgments, and other cognitive acts that manipulate information in working memory. (p. 653)

As humans evolved from earlier primates, and as our brains became progressively larger, most of that growth was in this association cortex—this vast web of communication carried by progressively longer and progressively more dense groups of axons. It is this axonal network that gives humans the capacity to process information in increasingly complex ways, including the capacity to store input in memory and to recall it quickly and efficiently when needed. Buckner and Krienen also point out that our dendritic connections within local cortical areas are more dense than those of other primates and that the continued development of these dendritic connections in areas such as the prefrontal cortex takes longer in the maturation process of humans. It is the association cortex that principally differentiates us from our primate relatives.

Rather than a chimpanzee, let us instead consider the development of the brain of a large mammal such as the giraffe. When a baby giraffe is born, it is capable of standing and walking (perhaps even running) within a few hours of birth. If it were not able to do this, it could easily fall prey to predators in the area. In order to optimize the giraffe's chances of survival, the sensory cortices, the motor cortex, and the associative cortex that links them together to create muscular movement and balance must be fully developed. The neurons are all in place, and they are all ready to carry messages that allow the infant giraffe to get up and walk.

Human infants, on the other hand, require months before they are capable of standing and walking. The cellular components of the human infant's brain have not matured to the same extent as the giraffe at the time of birth. There is a good reason this is so. Given the vastly increased size of the human brain in relation to other mammals and primates, if the human infant were to remain in the mother's womb until all its neural connections had matured, the infant's head would by then be too large to make it through the birth canal of the human female's pelvis. The process of labor and delivery for human women is already difficult enough, given the relatively narrow size of the birth canal. It often takes hours of contractions of the uterus and surrounding musculature to squeeze the infant's head through and then out of the birth canal. Thus humans are born with a brain that is not as far along in its cellular development as the brains of other mammals. This is a fundamental concept that we will discuss in greater depth in the next chapter, which addresses the development of human cognition.

The molecular biology of nerve conduction and neuronal myelination

We have explored how the various forms of neurons develop in the human brain, but we have left unanswered how it is that nerves carry out their fundamental activity: transmitting an electrochemical impulse from one place to another. As a first step in this discussion, let us consider how a metal wire carries out this function as part of an electrical system.

Much like axons, wires are long, thin chemical structures, typically made of an elemental metal such as copper. Copper is an especially efficient electrical conductor because of its atomic structure. Surrounding its positively charged nucleus, a copper atom has a collection of 29 negatively charged electrons. Of these, 28 are packed into orbital rings that bind them tightly to the nucleus. The 29th electron is in an outer orbital ring, all by itself. As such, it is more loosely bound, which allows it to connect to other atoms around it. Now picture a long, thin wire made of copper, as illustrated in figure 8.9.

If an electron from outside the wire enters the wire at one end, it can easily displace the free electron of a nearby copper atom. The electron that is displaced will then move to an

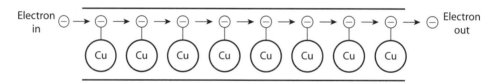

FIGURE 8.9 Electrical Conduction through a Copper Wire

adjacent atom and displace its electron. This sequence of electron movement from one copper atom to an adjacent atom will continue until it reaches the end of the wire, at which point a free electron will be in a position to move to an adjacent object. If that adjacent object happens to be our finger, we may feel an electrical shock. If it is another wire or similar substance, the electrical current generated in the wire will be passed on and will move through the new conductor. This is how electricity is transmitted from one end of a wire to the other.

The axon of a brain neuron is also a long, thin chemical structure. Rather than being made up of a single element such as copper, it is made up of a complex series of three-dimensional biochemical molecules. I illustrate the structure of a brain neuron in figure 8.10.

Surrounding the neuron is a cell membrane that controls, through biochemical processes, what gets into the cell and what goes out of the cell. In its resting state, the neuron has used these biochemical processes to push extra sodium ions to the outer surface of the cell membrane. These ions are positively charged (the reverse of the negative charge of the electrons in a copper wire) and thus create a cross-membrane difference in potential (difference in electrical charge), with the inner aspects of the neuron negatively charged. This separation of charges is referred to as the polarization of the cell membrane.

The laws of physics would suggest that the positively charged sodium ions on the outer surface of the cell would move across the cell membrane to the inner aspect of the cell so as to balance off the negative charge there—to "depolarize." The cell membrane, however, pre-

vents this from happening—that is, until it receives a chemical signal on one end. (This chemical signal is in the form of molecules called neurotransmitters whose specific function is to transmit impulses from one neuron to another. I discuss this transmission process below.) Once the neuron receives that signal, the cell membrane along its length depolarizes, allowing a sequential cascade of sodium ions to flow across the membrane to the interior of the cell until it reaches the end of the neuron and triggers the release of neurotransmitters to the adjacent neuron.

There is one additional aspect of the transmission of an impulse along the course of an axon that we should understand, as it comes up repeatedly in discussions we will have about the development of cognitive function in children—a topic covered in chapter 9. As described above, the outer surface of a neuronal axon is comprised of a cell membrane that selectively allows certain substances to cross it. In much the same way that copper wires that carry electricity are typically covered with a layer of insulating material to allow electrical conduction to take place more efficiently, the brain wraps the axon of a neuron in a biochemical insulating material called myelin.

Recall from our discussion above that when the nervous system begins the process of differentiation in the early phases of embryonic development, embryonic stem cells change into neural stem cells, which further differentiate into two types of cells: the neuroblasts, which become neurons, and glial precursor cells. Rather than participating directly in the transmission of information, these glial cells exist adjacent to

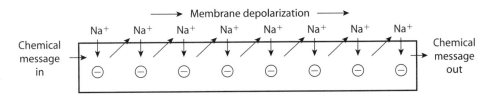

FIGURE 8.10. Impulse Conduction through a Neuron

the neurons, carrying out functions that support the neurons. In the case of axons, it is these glial cells that respond to the regular transmission of signals along an axon by attaching to the outer surface of the axon and gradually wrapping the axon in a fatty substance we call myelin. The specialized type of glial cell that performs this function is called an oligodendrocyte. If the functioning of these oligodendrocytes is impaired, the process of axon myelination will also be impaired as a result. Infants born extremely prematurely (before 32 weeks of gestation) are at risk of developing a form of brain injury called diffuse white matter injury, which can result in chronic impairment of brain functioning. Using a model of a similar brain injury in mice, Scafidi et al. (2013) showed that this type of injury to the white matter is due to impaired production of a growth factor that acts to stimulate the growth of oligodendrocytes and as a result the axonal myelination process. They administered this growth factor

to mice whose brains had undergone a form of injury similar to that caused by prematurity in humans and as a result were able to reverse the impact on oligodendrocyte functioning. The process of axon myelination in humans is illustrated in figure 8.11.

In response to biochemical signals given off by the axon as part of the transmission of impulses along its length, the oligodendrocytes begin to wrap sheets of myelin around the axon. The more regular the transmission of signals along the axon, the thicker the myelin sheath applied by the oligodendrocytes. Note, though, that the myelin sheath is not continuous along the length of the axon. It is interrupted at regular intervals by small segments, ranging in length from 0.2 to 2 millimeters, in which the axon is not covered by the myelin. These segments are referred to as the nodes of Ranvier. These nodes allow the transmission of the electrical impulse to proceed much more rapidly down the length of a neuron. Imagine a copper wire that gener-

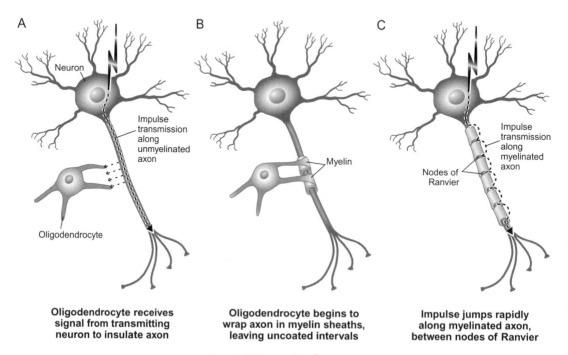

Oligodendrocyte receives signal from transmitting neuron to insulate axon

Oligodendrocyte begins to wrap axon in myelin sheaths, leaving uncoated intervals

Impulse jumps rapidly along myelinated axon, between nodes of Ranvier

FIGURE 8.11. Axon Myelination

ated a spark on its surface, with that spark jumping down a length of the wire, thus generating another spark that would also jump down the wire. In essence, this is what the nodes of Ranvier do. Rather than proceeding continuously down the entire length of the neuron, depolarization of the membrane can jump from node to node, bypassing the axonal segments that have been myelinated. Thus the conduction of the nerve impulse along a myelinated axon will happen much more rapidly than along a comparable axon that has not been myelinated.

Yeatman et al. (2014) studied the role of axonal myelination in the observed changes in brain structure and function from childhood through old age. They determined that "The myelination process is determined both by intrinsic genetic codes and extrinsic environmental factors. The level of electrical activity of an axon influences myelination, meaning that the myelination process is modified through experience." Explaining the role of myelination in facilitating communication between different cortical areas in the brain, they described how "Myelination speeds signal conduction between distant cortical regions and . . . determines the rate, quantity and nature of signals that a pathway transmits" (p. 8). As we will see when we discuss the neurobiological processes involved in learning, this process of myelination plays a crucial role.

Transmission of a nerve impulse across the synapse

As described above, the development of the human brain involves the proliferation of massive numbers of neurons (estimated to be in the billions) and the connection of these neurons through a complex web of axons and dendrites. The process of membrane depolarization we have just described conducts an impulse along the length of a single neuron. The question of how that impulse was triggered, and where it goes after it reaches the end of the neuron, involves a different set of chemical reactions. The synapse is the space in which two or more nerve cells adjoin each other. As shown in figure 8.12, the shapes of the cell membranes at their tips have adapted to this connection, with the end of one cell shaped optimally to transmit an impulse (referred to as the presynaptic button) and the other shaped to receive the chemical messengers transmitting that impulse.

In 2013, three scientists—James E. Rothman, Randy W. Schekman, and Thomas C. Südhof—were awarded the Nobel Prize in Physiology or Medicine "for their discoveries of machinery regulating vesicle traffic, a major transport system in our cells" (Nobel Assembly 2013). These scientists identified the precise biochemical structures and substances that transmit an impulse from one cell to another. They described small bubbles, called vesicles, containing key protein molecules called neurotransmitters. These vesicles lie adjacent to the inner aspect of the cell membrane. As shown in figure 8.12, when depolarization reaches the presynaptic button, the vesicles fuse with the cell membrane and then develop a small opening into the synaptic space between the cells, through which they emit their contents into the space. The membrane of the adjacent cell has specialized sensors called receptors that respond to the presence of neurotransmitters by triggering a new depolarization sequence along its membrane. Once the signal has been transmitted in this way, the vesicles reform inside the button to await the next impulse.

The process of transmission of the impulse across the synaptic space can take place dozens of times a second. As an impulse is transmitted repeatedly between the cells, the transmission process can become even more rapid, with increased amounts of neurotransmitters and heightened sensitivity of the adjacent receptors. These processes are important aspects of our ability to learn, which we will discuss at some length in chapter 9.

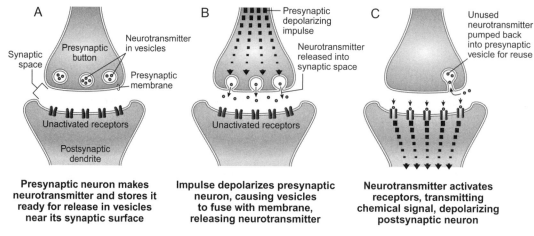

A

Synaptic space

Presynaptic button

Neurotransmitter in vesicles

Presynaptic membrane

Unactivated receptors

Postsynaptic dendrite

B

Presynaptic depolarizing impulse

Neurotransmitter released into synaptic space

Unactivated receptors

C

Unused neurotransmitter pumped back into presynaptic vesicle for reuse

Presynaptic neuron makes neurotransmitter and stores it ready for release in vesicles near its synaptic surface

Impulse depolarizes presynaptic neuron, causing vesicles to fuse with membrane, releasing neurotransmitter

Neurotransmitter activates receptors, transmitting chemical signal, depolarizing postsynaptic neuron

FIGURE 8.12. The Transmission of a Nerve Impulse across the Synapse

Brain systems for emotion and response to stress

The final aspect of brain structure and function I would like to discuss is those parts of the brain involved in sensing and responding to emotion and perceived stress. The various cortical areas we have discussed so far are largely involved in conscious activities such as listening, seeing, language, and movement. There is another set of brain structures and connections that underlies these cortical areas.

As described above, Broca's area receives input from a number of different cortical areas involved in language and integrates them to facilitate the learning and expression of language. In an analogous manner, the amygdala is the area of the brain that receives input from a number of areas of the brain and integrates this information into what we perceive as emotion. The amygdala is located adjacent to the hippocampus, in the frontal portion of the temporal lobe on either side of the brain. Emotions perceived by the amygdala can be triggered by sensing external stimuli, by remembering past experiences, or by a combination of the two. As part of this sensory process the amygdala has close connections to both the hippocampus and the thalamus.

The hippocampus is a section of the brain involved in storing memories of past events and retrieving them in response to certain related stimuli. The thalamus is a key part of our sensory apparatus that operates mostly at a subconscious level. It receives sensory input from our eyes and ears as well as from the sensory nerves of the body that come through the spinal cord, simultaneous with that information going to the sensory cortices. The thalamus is connected to the prefrontal cortex, which allows the brain to interpret those inputs in the context of conscious awareness and memory stored in the hippocampus. If we interpret those inputs as a threat, that message is conveyed to the amygdala, resulting in a feeling of fear or other related emotion.

This circuit takes time to respond to stimuli. Accordingly the thalamus also has a more rapid, direct link to the amygdala, so that certain stimuli will trigger an immediate response. Thus, we can be startled by something we hear or something we see, even before we are consciously aware of what is going on. Being startled in this way often triggers a physiological response encompassing pounding of the heart and associated feelings we are all familiar with. In generating this startle reflex the thalamus has a closely related unit, the hypothalamus, that is located directly below it and generates our physiological response to perceiving fear or being startled.

The hypothalamus is a major part of the unconscious control mechanism that maintains what is referred to as homeostasis. Homeostasis includes such functions as hunger and thirst, fatigue and the circadian rhythm of sleep, and our stress response. Another key aspect of homeostasis is thermostasis—the maintenance of a constant body temperature. The human body functions optimally when the internal body temperature is maintained at approximately 37 degrees Celsius. If our body temperature begins to drop, we feel cold, and our muscles sometimes shiver, contracting regularly and involuntarily so as to generate heat. If our temperature starts to rise due to a hot environment, we feel hot and begin to perspire. The evaporation from the skin of that perspiration cools us down. In these ways the hypothalamus helps maintain thermostasis.

The hypothalamus also helps to maintain allostasis—the process of maintaining an optimal physiologic stress response, appropriate for the level stress we perceive. The hypothalamus can respond in two ways. It can send messages directly over our autonomic (involuntary) nervous system to affected organs. Alternatively, it can respond by sending hormonal messages, referred to as releasing factors, to the pituitary gland, which in turn sends hormonal messages through the blood stream to the adrenal gland, located adjacent to the kidney. The adrenal gland responds to these messages by secreting three key hormones into the blood stream: epinephrine and norepinephrine (often referred to as adrenaline and noradrenaline), which produce a very rapid response, and cortisol (often referred to as cortisone), which produces a slower but more sustained response. The pounding of our heart and the rapid pulse we feel when we are startled is in response to the production of epinephrine and norepinephrine.

Our more general level of stress is often in response to the circulating level of cortisol. We need certain low levels of these hormones in our bloodstream when we are not sensing stress and increased levels when we are. The maintenance of these hormonal levels appropriate to our perceived level of stress is referred to as allostasis. The actual level of these circulating hormones is our allostatic load. The system of perception and response that generates these hormonal responses is referred to as the hypothalamic-pituitary-adrenal axis, or HPA axis for short.

As I described above in comparing a baby giraffe with a human infant, a central feature that distinguishes the human from the giraffe is the level of development of the systems of communication among the various structural components of the brain. At the time of their birth both a baby giraffe and a human infant have the basic structural components of the brain: the visual cortex, the auditory cortex, the sensory cortex, and the motor cortex, and the structures responsible for homeostasis and stress response. What have not yet developed in the human infant are the communications linkages among these various components. The axonal connections of the human have not matured and have a relatively low level of myelination. Similarly, the connections among the portions of the brain responsible for emotion and stress response have not matured. These communications linkages will develop and mature as the infant grows and matures.

This maturation process leaves open a period in which the development of neuronal communications can be affected by the physical and emotional environment in which the human infant is raised. Depending on the nature of those experiences, the neural communication mechanisms can develop more or less effectively. Makinodan et al. (2012) studied the brains of newborn mice, some of which were isolated immediately after weaning and deprived of any adult attention. Compared to mice that had experienced nurturing, the level of oligo-dendrocyte activity and neuronal myelination was substantially lower in the deprived mice, suggesting that the surrounding environment can directly affect the development of neuronal communication. This aspect of brain development is often referred to as brain plasticity. In addition to the extent of axonal myelination, environmental influences can also affect the efficiency of the synaptic transmission mechanism described above. Studies of genetically identical human twins who were separated at birth and raised in different social environments have confirmed the importance of the plasticity of the brain.

A crucial issue we will discuss in future chapters is the extent to which this brain plasticity is a one-way process. If a child raised in stressful or otherwise disadvantaged circumstances develops weaker axonal myelination and synaptic transmission when compared to a child raised in a more nurturing environment, are those differences reversible? As described by Britto and Pérez-Escamilla, "during specific periods of development experiences have the ability to potentiate or inhibit neural connectivity . . . Theorists have argued that while children may not receive the required environmental inputs at the appropriate time and that this may hamper development they posit that this inability to develop is not permanent" (2013, p. 238). As we will see, there is a growing body of data indicating that the neural impacts of early adversity, often referred to as toxic stress, can be reversed through appropriate interventions.

A second related issue is the question of how long in the process of human development brain plasticity continues. Is the structure of the human brain fixed and unchangeable by adolescence or early adulthood? Alternatively, does the plasticity persist even into older age, though perhaps at a somewhat slower rate? Since the neural structure and processes of the human brain are largely responsible for patterns of human behavior, and human behavior is largely responsible for the level of well-being experienced by humans across the life course, fully understanding the extent of these effects is crucial to understanding how and when to intervene to address unhealthy or destructive behaviors.

Summary

Rather than being a single organ with one principal function, the human brain is a complex system of separate cortical areas, each involved in specific functions, connected by a complex web of axons. These differentiated cortical areas and associated neural connections develop from a common set of embryonic stem cells. While the cortical structure of the human brain has a great deal in common with other primates, it is the neural connections between these cortical areas that distinguish the human brain.

These connections depend on the efficient conveyance of the biochemical information of a nerve impulse along the neuron itself and between neurons at their many connections. The brain has developed ways to increase the efficiency of this transmission process in those neurons that are activated most frequently and to remove those neural connections that go unused. This concept of brain plasticity—of the cellular structure of the brain able to change over time in response to patterns of brain activity—is key to understanding the many ways that environmental factors can influence the structure and function of the human brain.

Now that we have gained a basic understanding of the way the human brain is structured and how the various structural components communicate among themselves, the next thing to look at is how the brain develops its awareness and understanding of the world in which we live. The American Psychological Association defines *cognition* as the "processes of knowing, including attending, remembering, and reasoning; also the content of the processes, such as concepts and memories." How the human infant develops these processes in response to both the prenatal uterine environment and the family environment into which it is born is a central aspect of the development of human behavior, and I address this topic in chapter 9.

REFERENCES

American Psychological Association. Glossary of psychological terms, available at www.apa.org/research/action/glossary.aspx, accessed 2/16/14.

Britto, P. R., & Pérez-Escamilla, R. 2013. No second chances? Early child experiences in human development. Social Science and Medicine 97: 238-40.

Buckner, R. L., & Krienen, F. M. 2013. The evolution of distributed association networks in the human brain. Trends in Cognitive Science 17(12): 648-65.

Congressional Budget Office. 2014. The budget and economic outlook: 2014 to 2024, available at www.cbo.gov/publication/45010, accessed 2/8/14.

Duboc, B. The growth cone. The Brain from Top to Bottom, available at http://thebrain.mcgill.ca, accessed 2/9/14.

Fernald, A., Marchman, V. A. , & Weisleder, A. 2013. SES differences in language processing skill and vocabulary are evident at 18 months. Developmental Science 16(2): 234-48.

Makinodan, M., Rosen, K. M., & Corfas, C. 2012. A critical period for social experience-dependent oligodendrocyte maturation and myelination. Science 337 (6100): 1357-60.

Moon, C., Lagercrantz, H., & Kuhl, P. K. 2013. Language experienced in utero affects vowel perception after birth: A two-country study. Acta Paediatrica 102(2): 156-60.

Nobel Assembly at Karolinska Institutet. The Nobel Prize in Physiology or Medicine 2013, available at www.nobelprize.org/nobel_prizes/medicine/laureates/2013/press.html, accessed 2/16/14.

Scafidi, J., Hammond, T. R., Scafidi, S., et al. 2013. Intranasal epidermal growth factor treatment rescues neonatal brain injury. Nature 506(7487): 230-4.

Who can my Marketplace information be shared with and why? Available at www.healthcare.gov/how-we-use-your-data/, accessed 2/2/14.

Yeatman, J. D., Wandell, B. A., & Mezer, A. A. 2014. Lifespan maturation and degeneration of human brain white matter. Nature Communications 5. doi:10.1038/ncomms5932.

CHAPTER 9

Cognition, Behavior,
and Well-Being

At the time of its birth, a human infant has already developed the basic components of its brain: the visual cortex, the auditory cortex, the sensory cortex, the motor cortex, and the structures responsible for homeostasis and stress response. What the human infant has not yet fully developed are the communications linkages among these various components that will enable them to function in a coordinated manner. While the axonal connections among the various functional cortices are largely present, they have not yet matured, due to a relatively low level of axonal myelination.

A news report describing the work of Carla Shatz and her colleagues at the Stanford Bio-X center describes the newborn human infant as "a data acquisition machine, absorbing information to finish honing the job of brain wiring that started before birth" (Adams 2014). In the previous chapter I used the structure of Internet sites such as Healthcare.gov as an analogy for the structure of the human brain. I described both as "a complex network of central information sources and interconnecting webs of communication." For the human infant, the central information sources are largely functional at birth, while the interconnecting communication webs are not. In order for the infant to begin the process of developing cognitive awareness and responses, the axonal interconnections connecting the functional cortices must become myelinated, thus allowing rapid and repeated communication between cortices that results in action.

This is not to say that the axonal connections in the infant brain at the time of birth are without any function. Evidence by Moon et al. (2014) suggests that newborn infants are capable of distinguishing vowel sounds from the language spoken by their mother from those sounds of another language (see chapter 8). Simply recognizing language-specific phonemes is not the same as acquiring language. That process will require repeated sensation of sounds spoken by another person (often the mother), the attachment of meaning to those sounds, and the ability (often through trial and error) to reproduce those sounds. When that process has begun to take effect, the infant will have begun to acquire language.

Hart and Risley (1995) studied 42 families with young children. Based on the parents' occupation, the families were approximately equally distributed across upper, middle, and lower socioeconomic status (SES). Starting when the children were 7-9 months old, they visited each family at home for an hour each month, directly observing and recording interactions between parents and children. After about two and a half years of these visits, they analyzed the data they had gathered.

By the time the children were 3 years old, the researchers identified clear trends in the amount of talk the children had been exposed to and the children's vocabulary growth. Children in lower-SES families both heard fewer words spoken by the adults in their household and were more likely to hear words the researchers described as prohibitions and discouragements rather than affirmatives and encouragements. The lower-SES children had smaller vocabularies than children of the same age from professional families as well as showing slower growth in vocabulary. The researchers then followed the children until they were aged 9 to 10 and found that the level of vocabulary demonstrated at age 3 was a strong predictor of scores on a range of vocabulary assessment instruments.

In chapter 8 we also discussed the work by Fernald et al. (2013) that studied language development in infants aged 18-24 months. They used the speed with which an infant could associate the sound of a spoken word with a picture of the object represented by the word as a measure of the extent of language development. In a study of English-learning infants from a broad socioeconomic range of families, they found that, at 18 months of age, infants recog-

nized an average vocabulary of 142 spoken words. They also found, however, a striking difference in that vocabulary level when comparing infants from lower-SES families with those from higher-SES families. At 18 months, higher-SES infants recognized an average of 174 words, while lower-SES infants recognized an average of 107 words. By 24 months of age, both groups had increased their vocabulary substantially, to 442 words for higher-SES infants and 288 words for lower-SES infants. At 24 months of age, the lower-SES children were already six months behind the higher-SES children in language development. As described by Fernald et al., "The infant who can interpret a familiar word more rapidly has more resources available for attending to subsequent words, with advantages for learning new words that come later in the sentence . . . Vocabulary knowledge also serves as a foundation for later literacy, and language proficiency in preschool is predictive of academic success" (2013, p. 244)

Weisleder and Fernald (2013) explored this issue further in a study of 19 lower-SES infants being raised in primarily Spanish-speaking families. When the infants were 19 months old, the researchers provided the parents with a sensitive audio recorder that was placed in the chest pocket of a lightweight jacket the infant wore. They recorded the sounds each child heard during one day. In analyzing the sound recordings, the researchers counted how many spoken words were directed at the child. When the children were 24 months old, the researchers used a standardized scale of vocabulary recognition to have the parents estimate how many words their infant both understood and was able to say. They found a significant association between the amount of child-directed speech and the child's spoken language ability. In discussing these findings, the authors commented that "differences in how quickly and reliably children interpret familiar words in real time reflect variability in a cognitive skill that facilitates further language learning . . . a critical step in the path from early language experience to later vocabulary knowledge is the influence of language exposure on infants' speech-processing skill" (p. 2149).

Festa et al. (2014) found that children from low-income, immigrant Hispanic families such as those studied by Weisleder and Fernald face an additional disadvantage in developing early language ability. In addition to speaking directly to children, sharing a book with a young child also helps children to develop language ability. In their study of families in California with young children, Festa et al. observed that immigrant Hispanic families showed the lowest frequency of sharing a book with their children on a daily basis—53.4 percent of children in Hispanic families as compared to 78.0 percent of non-Hispanic white children, with even lower rates (47.1 percent) for Hispanic children with both parents born outside the United States.

In chapter 8 I described the process through which an unmyelinated axon becomes myelinated through repetitive transmission of impulses along its length. It is this repetitive signaling from one cortical area to another along the connecting axons that triggers the myelination process and establishes the capacity for rapid communication between these areas. Recall also from figure 8.5 the different parts of the brain that are involved with the acquisition of and expression of language. Patterns of sound from the auditory cortex and images of sight from the visual cortex are integrated in Wernicke's area. As an infant repeatedly hears a word and sees the object or the action the word is intended to represent, that association is then stored in memory. At a later time the infant can hear the word without also seeing the image and, through the connection between the auditory cortex and Wernicke's area, retrieve from memory the image of the object the word represents. The more often this happens, the more efficient the communication link through Wernicke's area and the larger the vocabulary the child has available.

In a study on infant vocabulary, Fernald et al. played a recording of a woman's voice saying words such as *doggy, birdie, ball,* and *book.* They then showed a picture to one side of the infant of the object represented by the word and on the other side a picture of another object usually familiar to children but not related to the spoken word. They closely watched the direction of the child's gaze to see if, and how quickly, it focused on the object represented by the word. If a child quickly looked at the picture of a dog when hearing *doggy,* the researchers concluded that she or he had heard the word spoken while also looking at a dog on a repeated basis. The infant had likely myelinated the axons within the brain that connect the sound *doggy* to the visual image of a dog, such that the image could quickly be recalled when triggered by the sound. Fundamental learning had taken place, triggered by someone speaking to the child on a regular basis.

The development of cognition

The American Psychological Association defines the concept of cognition as the "processes of knowing, including attending, remembering, and reasoning; also the content of the processes, such as concepts and memories." It goes on to describe cognitive development as including, "imagining, perceiving, reasoning, and problem solving." In a similar manner, the *Oxford English Dictionary* defines cognition as including "knowledge, consciousness; acquaintance with a subject."

The infant who looked at the picture of the dog upon hearing *doggy* knew what a dog was. She or he had acquired early cognition. Throughout childhood, and no doubt continuing into adulthood, she or he will expand that cognition—that "knowing . . . attending, remembering, and reasoning." By high school, perhaps she or he will know a foreign language and will be able to calculate a regression equation if given the correlation and variance of two variables.

TABLE 9.1. The Stages of Cognitive Development as Proposed by Jean Piaget (1964)

Stage	Age	Cognitive development
Sensory-motor	Birth–2	Sense of self as separate Beginnings of language Object permanence
Preoperational	2–7	Symbolic meaning of words Expanded use of language Understands concept of numbers
Concrete operational	7–12	Classification and ordering of objects Logical reasoning Mathematical ability
Formal operational	12 and older	Able to reason hypothetically Understands abstract relationships Understands moral concepts

That level of cognition, of course, is at an entirely different stage than recognizing the word *doggy*.

Jean Piaget was a Swiss developmental psychologist who spent much of the 20th century studying how children acquire knowledge. He conducted a series of observations and experiments at his center in Geneva, published a number of books in the area, and developed a reputation as a leading scholar in the study of child development.

In 1964, Cornell University and the University of California, Berkeley, jointly sponsored coordinated conferences to discuss Piaget's work and the work of other leading scholars. Piaget developed an address summarizing his ideas on cognitive development in children and presented the address at both conferences. Piaget's address (1964), along with the other papers from the conference, was published in a special issue of the *Journal of Research in Science Teaching*. Piaget described what he considered to be four distinct stages in the cognitive development of children, as illustrated in table 9.1.

Piaget based his theory on the necessary sequencing of successive stages of cognitive development. These core concepts can only be learned as part of the maturation of the child's brain, through a combination of reflexive actions, development of motor coordination, realization that the outer world exists separately from the child itself, and learning about properties of physical objects. As described by Piaget, "learning is possible if you base the more complex structure on simpler structures, that is, when there is a natural relationship and development of structures" (1964, p. 184). The development of the core sensory-motor capabilities progresses as the child's experience with the outside world leads to the successive development of myelinated axonal connections between different parts of the brain.

Piaget described the first of these developmental stages as the "sensory-motor, pre-verbal stage, lasting approximately 18 months of life. During this stage is developed the practical knowledge which constitutes the substructure of later representational knowledge" (p. 177). By about age 2 the child has progressed into Piaget's second stage, the "preoperational" stage, in which a child develops "the beginnings of language, of the symbolic function, and therefore of thought, or representation" (p. 177). It is in this stage of development that a child begins to appreciate the symbolic nature of spoken and written words (*doggy* refers to that furry thing that licks me in the face and sometimes scares me when he barks). The child also learns basic numeric and spatial concepts that help to understand the broader world. Piaget described the experience of one of his adult colleagues, who as a child learned the concept of numbers. At about age 4 or 5, the colleague was sitting in his garden and playing with pebbles. He placed a series of pebbles in a straight line on the ground. He had by then learned his numbers, so he counted the pebbles from one end of the line to the other: 10 pebbles. He was fascinated to find that when he counted the pebbles in the reverse direction, he again counted 10 pebbles. He then placed the pebbles in a circle on the ground and counted them again. Again there were 10 pebbles! "Now indeed, what did he discover? He did not discover a property of pebbles; he discovered a property of the action of ordering. The pebbles had no order . . . He discovered that the sum was independent of the order" (p. 180).

The child had discovered that the number 10 exists independently of the pebbles. This allowed him to appreciate numbers as symbolic concepts and to explore their association with other numbers. Using this symbolic understanding, he will be able to learn that "two plus two equals four" and to transfer this specific understanding into his memory through a process of axonal myelination similar to the process of learning what *doggy* means. This will have substantial importance when, later in this chapter, we discuss Daniel Kahneman's concept of "thinking fast and thinking slow."

In the third stage of cognitive development, from about age 7 through age 11, what Piaget describes as "concrete operations" begin to appear. These concrete operations are compared to "formal" operations that occur in his fourth developmental stage. Examples of concrete operations described by Piaget include "classification, ordering . . . spatial and temporal operations, and all the fundamental operations of elementary logic" (p. 177). At this stage children begin to be able to learn, understand, and use concepts from mathematics and science.

In the last stage described by Piaget, beginning at about the age of 11 or 12, "the child reaches the level of what I call formal or hypothetic-deductive operations; that is, he can now reason on hypotheses, and not only on objects" (p. 177). It is only in this stage that children begin to be able to understand complex mathematical concepts, such as probabilities, and abstract moral concepts, such as social justice.

In summarizing his four stages of cognitive development, Piaget underscores the importance of the developing biologic organism that sets human aside from other species. It is the unique capacities of the human brain that allow this type of learning to progress throughout childhood and adolescence. We are continuously exposed to stimuli from our environment, and we develop patterns of response to those stimuli. As Piaget explained in his address to the 1964 conferences, "I would propose that above all, between the stimulus and the response, there is the organism, the organism and its structures. The stimulus is really a stimulus only when it is assimilated into a structure and it is the structure which sets off the response" (p. 182).

The development of language and reading ability as examples of Piaget's stages of development

Piaget based the timing of his proposed stages of development on the developmental process in a child's brain. This principle is illustrated in the manner in which children first learn language and subsequently learn to read. These stages in cognitive development parallel the stages in the development of the neural connections in the brain of the growing child.

As described in chapter 8, the process of language development depends on the development of neural connections between the gray matter sections of the brain responsible for two of the core senses: hearing and vision. In order to develop language, an infant must first develop myelinated neural connections between the auditory cortex (sensing the sound of the word), the visual cortex (sensing the visual image represented by that sound), the cortical area that integrates these two sensory inputs as language (Wernicke's area), and the area in the frontal lobe responsible for storing in memory the meaning of words based on the learned association between those sensations (Broca's area).

Infants begin to develop this process in the first few months of life by recognizing spoken words, based on the repetitive hearing of specific sounds and seeing their associated images. By the age of 18-24 months, they begin to understand a substantial vocabulary of words, which they in turn learn to speak. The more they are spoken to directly, the larger their vocabulary. As described by Fernald et al., "Variability among individuals in verbal abilities is influenced to some extent by genetic factors, but the contributions of early experience to differences in language proficiency are also substantial" (2013, p. 243).

Piaget described this early period, from birth to about 18 months of age, as the sensory-motor stage. During this time the basic cognitive processes and neural structures necessary for acquiring language are being developed. Until they are developed, infants are not able to express language. He describes the next stage, beginning at about 18-24 months of age and lasting until about age 7, as the preoperational stage. In this stage the child has begun the development of verbal language and is now capable of building the ability to read, which is essentially the next stage in the full development of language.

This brings up an interesting question. As children transition from the sensory-motor stage, where they have begun the process of language development, to the preoperational stage, where they can expand on this ability in both the spoken and the written word, will their initial level of verbal capacity at age 18-24 months be associated with their reading ability at age 7 years? Fernald et al. suggest these levels of development will be associated. "Vocabulary knowledge also serves as a foundation for later literacy, and language proficiency in preschool is predictive of academic success . . . Differences among children in language growth established by 3 years of age tend to persist and are predictive of later school success or failure" (pp. 244-5).

In their article "Learning to See Words" (2012), Wandell et al. describe our increasing understanding of the functional and structural aspects of brain activity involved in transitioning from understanding spoken language to understanding written language, that is, learning to read. In order to read, a child must be able rapidly to recognize words on a page and to associate those visual images with the meaning of the word learned through the earlier acquisition of spoken language. As described by the authors, "to read a child must develop adequate visual acuity and learn to understand speech. Competence at these tasks is predictive of future reading: Children who are efficient at hearing and manipulating the sounds of speech are usually good at learning to read" (p. 32).

Wandell and colleagues go on to describe recent advances in brain imaging that measure the effectiveness of the communication among areas of the brain involved with vision and with verbal language. Researchers have identified specific white-matter structures that interconnect these various areas of the brain to enable reading. One of the most important of these axonal connections is the arcuate fasciculus (AF), which connects Wernicke's area to Broca's area, as described in chapter 8.

Yeatman et al. (2012) studied how early reading ability is reflected in children's neural structures. In introducing the research, Yeatman underscores the importance of neural connections such as the AF, describing how "Reading requires efficient communication within a network of visual, auditory, and language-processing regions that are separated by many centimeters. Hence, the white-matter fascicles that connect these regions are critical for proficient reading" (p. E3045).

Yeatman's team followed a total of 39 children between the ages of 7 and 12. All were native speakers of English. Over a period of three years the researchers administered three sequential MRI brain scans to each of the children. They also administered sequential assessment of reading skills and associated cognitive skills. They then evaluated the change over time in the structure of the AF, comparing students who were strong readers with those who were weak readers. They found an interesting pattern of change in the AF as the two groups of children got older.

Using a measure of axonal structure called fractional anisotropy, the researchers found that between the ages of 7 and 12, the functional efficiency of the AF changed. For children who at age 7 were strong readers, that efficiency increased in a linear pattern, while for children who were weak readers at age 7, it decreased over time. Yeatman et al. explained this by suggesting that the axons in the AF were becoming increasingly myelinated in the stronger readers, while in the weaker readers some of the neurons were becoming myelinated while others were being "pruned" due to relative inactivity. "The myelination process is plastic; the level of electrical activity of an axon influences myelination . . . During development, some axons grow, and other axons are eliminated in a process called 'pruning' . . . Underused axons are pruned away during childhood, and the remaining axons are increasingly myelinated" (p. 3049).

Recall that the infant brain has many more axons than it will eventually need as the brain matures into adulthood. This creates a "use it or lose it" situation: axons that are used repeatedly to connect cortical areas become myelinated, thereby becoming much more efficient and available for reuse when called on, while the axons that aren't called on to carry messages may eventually be removed from the brain. This seems to suggest that, just as hearing more spoken words improves the word recognition of infants aged 18-24 months, reading more words between ages 7 and 12 makes children better readers. As Yeatman describes, "Variation in the quality of early-life language input, the differential effects of children's reading experience, the timing of instruction with respect to these processes, and genetic factors could all contribute [to the development of reading ability]" (p. 3050).

This makes intuitive sense—the better the child is at reading, the more reading that child will do. The more reading a child does over time, the better that child becomes at reading. Again as described by Yeatman, "The rate at which a child learns to read early in elementary school is highly predictive of the person's relative reading proficiency throughout childhood, adolescence, and adulthood" (p. 3051). Growing up in a situation of socioeconomic disadvantage or having poorly educated parents who don't speak as much or read as much to their children can affect a child's development of language and his or her subsequent development of reading ability. These effects can be reflected in weakened white-matter communication ability in key areas of the brain and may stay with the child as he or she grows through adolescence and into adulthood.

Lonigan et al. describe the development of literacy as an "emergent process" that begins early in the child's life and continues throughout the various stages of development. "An emergent literacy approach departs from other perspectives on reading acquisition in suggesting that there is no clear demarcation between reading and prereading . . . Significant sources of individual differences in later reading skills are present prior to school entry" (2000, p. 596). This brings up a key point regarding the development of cognitive abilities. Just as the process of developing literacy is a continuous one, encompassing early childhood through the early school years, that process continues as the child progresses through adolescence and into adulthood. The same level of brain plasticity that allowed the strong reader at age 7 to develop even more myelinated axons in the AF by age 9 will also allow the relatively weak reader at age 7 to grow into a strong reader, with increasingly myelinated AF axons, *if* she or he has the opportunity and the motivation to invest time and energy in becoming a better reader.

Learning math in Piaget's next stage

As conceptualized by Piaget, once a child has developed language and has begun to understand the symbolic nature of many learned concepts, she or he is ready to move on to the concrete operations stage, learning "the operations of classification, ordering, the construction of the idea of number, . . . and all the fundamental operations . . . of elementary mathematics, of elementary geometry, and even of elementary physics" (Piaget 1964, p. 177). This stage generally spans the years between ages 7 and 12.

Is there a section of the brain that responds to numbers, in a way similar to the response to verbal and written language? Shum et al. (2013) addressed this question in a study of seven adults between the ages of 24 and 48. Rather than brain MRI scans, they used electrodes fastened to the scalp that measured underlying brain wave activity. Subjects were shown an array of images of numbers, letters, and mixtures of both. By comparing patterns of brain activity to the image shown, researchers identified a specific area in the temporal lobe of the brain that was close to, but distinct from, the parts of the brain involved in language and reading. The authors commented that "This anatomical proximity is important because the two sites are frequently coengaged in visual processing of words and numbers that co-occur frequently in our everyday life" (p. 6714). They go on to

point out, however, that their separate locations may account for those individuals who may be very skilled in mathematics, but less skilled in reading (or vice versa).

Do children undergo a continual process of neuronal development that results in later mathematical ability, analogous to the process of developing language and reading skills? Will there be stronger axonal myelination in the brain areas responsible for processing numbers in those children who exhibit stronger mathematical skills in school? Supekar et al. (2013) studied the effects of a targeted math tutoring program in 24 third-grade children aged 8-9. The tutoring program emphasized conceptual instruction and practice in rapid retrieval of mathematical facts. They measured math ability before and after the eight-week tutoring program and compared these results to those of 16 other third-graders who had not participated in the tutoring sessions. In addition to the testing of math skills, all the children in the study had a series of other assessments at the beginning of the study, including IQ testing, overall academic assessment, and behavioral assessment. Each child, both in the study group and in the control group, also underwent a functional MRI study of the brain.

Perhaps not surprisingly, the math skills of the children participating in the tutoring program increased significantly, while the skills of the control group did not change. The researchers then looked to see whether any of the pretutoring assessments was associated with the level of increase in math skills each child showed as a result of the tutoring. None of the behavioral measures, including the IQ testing, was associated with a child's increase in math ability. The researchers did find, however, a significant association between certain brain structural components shown on the MRI and the increase in math ability. In particular, they noted a strong association between the increase in math skills, the volume of the gray matter in the right hippocampus, and the white-matter connections between the hippocampus and the prefrontal cortex. The authors concluded, "Our findings suggest that arithmetic skill acquisition during this early period of learning depends on the integrity of hippocampal-prefrontal cortex and hippocampal-basal ganglia functional circuits. Children who exhibited higher intrinsic functional connectivity in these circuits before tutoring showed the greatest performance improvement in math problem solving" (p. 8234).

In a process that closely parallels the development of language and reading, the development of mathematical skills is based on certain types of repetitive instructional activities, which are associated with cellular changes in neural gray matter and the axonal connections between different brain cortices. Consistent with Piaget's views, math skills develop at a somewhat later stage in the development process than language skills. Similarly, the development of basic skills in arithmetic builds a foundation on which children can develop higher-level math skills that involve abstract reasoning and rules of logic in addition to basic computational skills.

We have seen that lower socioeconomic status is associated with slower development of language skills in children aged 18-24 months and that subsequent reading ability is closely associated with the earlier development of language. While the Supekar study does not address this question explicitly, it is reasonable to expect a child's socioeconomic status also to be associated with the development of early mathematical skills. In a study commissioned by the National Academy of Sciences titled *From Neurons to Neighborhoods*, Shonkoff and Phillips report that, "From birth to age 5, children rapidly develop foundational capabilities on which subsequent development builds . . . Striking disparities in what children know and can do are evident well before they enter kindergarten. These differences are strongly associated with social and economic circumstances, and they

are predictive of subsequent academic performance" (2000, p. 5).

In proposing his stages of cognitive development, Piaget is clear that the physical maturation of the child's body, especially the nervous system, is a principal determinant of how these developmental stages progress. In his 1964 talk, he explained the sequential development of the four stages in the following way.

> What factors can be called upon to explain the development from one set of [cognitive] structures to another? It seems to me that there are four main factors: first of all *maturation* . . . , since this development is a continuation of embryogenesis; second, the role of *experience* of the effects of the physical environment on the structures of intelligence; third, *social transmission* in the broad sense (linguistic transmission, education, etc.); and fourth, a factor which is too often neglected but one which seems to me fundamental and even the principal factor. I shall call this the factor of *equilibration* or if you prefer it, of self-regulation. (p. 178)

Piaget identifies many of the same factors we now recognize as influencing the early physical and cognitive development of the child. He describes the interaction between genetically driven physical maturation, the quality of the family environment, the impact of the social environment, and the child's development of the ability to self-regulate as key to understanding the stages of cognitive development.

Piaget acknowledged the limited scientific understanding at that time of neural structure at the cellular and molecular level. As he described it in 1964, "we know practically nothing about the maturation of the nervous system beyond the first months of the child's existence" (p. 178). Nonetheless he appreciated the important role the environment plays on nervous system maturation. He seems to be describing the groundwork for our current understanding of the impact on neural structure of the family and social environment, through the process we now refer to as epigenetic imprinting—the influence of factors in the environment external to the child on how the child's genes are expressed, without actually changing the molecular structure of those genes, during the process of growth and maturation.

Recent advances in developmental neuroscience have provided some new evidence in support of Piaget's concept of staged development. We have come to appreciate that there are certain periods during early child development, referred to as critical periods, during which the child is most susceptible to epigenetic influences. Some of the most crucial of these critical periods occur in the first several months after birth, when a child fine-tunes his or her physiologic response to stress and begins the process of language development.

Not everyone agrees with Piaget's conceptualization of the stages of cognitive development. An early-20th-century Russian psychologist, Lev Vygotsky, suggested that child development was much more dependent on the interaction between the child and his or her environment, which he called the "Zone of Proximal Development." In a 1978 translation of his earlier essays published between 1930 and 1934, Vygotsky described this zone as "the distance between the actual development level as determined by independent problem solving and the level of potential development as determined through problem solving under adult guidance or in collaboration with our capable peers" (p. 86). As seen by Vygotsky, children's emotional and cognitive development is powerfully influenced by the interaction with adults and peers around them. The better the quality of that interaction, the more rapidly the child's development can progress. From this perspective, a child's developmental stages are more variable in timing than those proposed by Piaget.

Clark and Chalmers (1998) go one step further, suggesting that the human mind is not limited to what happens in the brain. Rather, the mind "extends" to include physical objects in the environment as a central part of the cognitive process. In describing their "extended mind" theory, they offer two popular games as examples: Tetris and Scrabble. In Tetris, a computer game released in the 1980s, the player must rapidly rotate and move horizontally geometric images on a computer screen in order to fit them into the appropriately shaped location. Clark and Chalmers suggest that doing this mental process of rotation and movement without the help of the computer would take substantially longer than the same process using the computer. Similarly, having a set of Scrabble tiles displayed to look at and rearrange allows one to identify words spelled by those tiles much more rapidly than having to do the same process in the unaided mind. They refer to these actions as "epistemic" actions that "alter the world so as to aid and augment cognitive processes" (1998, p. 8). In a sense, the Tetris screen and the Scrabble tiles are simple extensions of the human mind. Describing the use of Scrabble tiles, they suggest that "In a very real sense, the re-arrangement of the tiles on the tray is not part of action; it is part of *thought*" (p. 10). Whether in acts of memory, the use of language, or something as simple as using a Google map to find the location of the Museum of Modern Art in New York City, "cognition is often taken to be continuous with processes in the environment . . . all sorts of processes beyond the borders of consciousness play a crucial role in cognitive processing" (p. 10).

Memory and its role in cognition

By now it should be evident that much of the process of cognitive development depends on the capacity to remember. Memory is involved in infants' associating certain sounds they hear with images they see. It is also involved in learning to connect the visual images of words on the page of a book with the meaning and implications of those words. Memory comes in more than one shape and size. By means of example, consider some texts I have memorized as part of my mentoring of the college students I work with and the steps I take to remember what I was planning to purchase when I go to the grocery store.

Often, when a student meets with me to discuss her or his efforts at writing a research paper or research report, I will hand her or him a printed copy of the following, and then recite it to them from memory: *Four score and seven years ago our fathers brought forth on this continent a new nation, conceived in liberty, and dedicated to the proposition that all men are created equal . . .*

After reciting this, I ask the students to identify the thesis sentence in Lincoln's address at Gettysburg. Many students aren't aware of why Lincoln traveled to Gettysburg to give the address. I explain the importance for the North of the Battle of Gettysburg and the symbolic significance of the dedication of the new national cemetery located on the site of the battlefield. I then point out that the thesis sentence—*We have come to dedicate a portion of that field, as a final resting place for those who here gave their lives that that nation might live*—is embedded in the middle of the text, preceded by an explanation of the historical context of the battle and followed by the implications for future action of the sacrifices made on that battlefield.

Other students come to me for advice about life choices they are facing. Should they go to medical school, or should they go to public health school? Should they be science majors or humanities majors? I also hand these students a printed copy and begin to recite from memory:

Two roads diverged in a yellow wood,
And sorry I could not travel both
And be one traveler, long I stood . . .

I emphasize for the students that, even though the final lines of the poem say *I took the one less traveled by, / And that has made all the difference,* the title of the poem is "The Road Not Taken." It turns out there wasn't a less-traveled road. After initially glancing at both roads, Frost realized:

Though as for that the passing there
Had worn them really about the same,
And both that morning equally lay
In leaves no step had trodden black.

If you have ever seen a Vermont leaf fall in the autumn, you know what the woods look like before any feet have had a chance to turn the yellow leaves to black.

So, I guess I might say that I have a fairly good memory, as I usually am able to recite either of these on short notice, including words, timing, and emphasis. Yet if you were ever to come with me to the grocery store, you might question the strength of my memory. If I need to buy three things that day, I can remember them and be fairly assured that when I walk out of the store, each will be in my bag. If I need four things, I have learned to make a list. Otherwise I'll typically remember three of the four and get home not being able to remember what the fourth one was.

Why can I recite from memory Robert Frost's "The Road Not Taken" and Abraham Lincoln's Gettysburg Address, but I can't remember the fourth thing I was supposed to buy? Because there is more than one type of memory! Squire and Zola have described these as "declarative memory . . . the capacity for conscious recollection of facts and events" and "nondeclarative memory . . . a heterogeneous collection of nonconscious learning capacities that are expressed through performance" (1996, p. 13515). By their definition I am attempting to use declarative memory when I go to the grocery store without a list and nondeclarative memory when I recite Lincoln or Frost for my students.

Swedish neuroscientist Torkel Klinberg refers to these as "long term memory and working memory. The long term memory is the memory system that stores learned facts, rules, names and experiences. It's the memory that stores what we traditionally associate with learning at school . . . Working memory, on the other hand, keeps information up front just when we need it and holds relevant items 'in our head' when we're solving a problem" (2013, p. x).

Psychologist Daniel Kahneman refers to these as "System 1" memory and "System 2" memory. He describes them in the following terms:

- *System 1* operates automatically and quickly, with little or no effort and no sense of voluntary control.
- *System 2* allocates attention to the effortful mental activities that demand it, including complex computations (2011, p. 20).

When I recite a Robert Frost poem from memory, I am relying on System 1; when I try to remember what to buy at the store, I am invoking System 2.

Do I have a good memory (reciting poems from memory) or do I have a weak memory (only being able to remember three things to buy)? It seems I am perfectly normal in both. Klinberg suggests that it is typical for adults to be able to keep only about four items in working memory, which means that at my functional capacity of three shopping items (at least when confronted by the multiple distractions of the grocery store) isn't so far off.

Kahneman refers to these two mnemonic (i.e., having to do with memory) processes in another way that seems intuitively useful. As the title of his book suggests, he also refers to System 1 as "thinking fast" and System 2 as "thinking slow." He provides an instructive example of these two modes of memory (p. 20). He asks us to find the answer to the following two mathematical expressions:

$$2+2$$

$$17 \times 24$$

We all know that two plus two equals four. We learned that sometime in our childhood, and it has stayed within our System 1 memory since then. We don't actually need to do a mathematical computation. The entire phrase of "two plus two equals four" is stored within our brain cells, ready for us to call on when prompted.

On the other hand, to calculate 17×24, I can close my eyes and try to go through the steps I learned in school ("7 times 4 is 28, put down the 8 and carry the 2 . . ."), or I can use one of the extended mind tools Clark and Chalmers suggest are part of the cognitive process, such as a pencil and paper or a calculator. To do any of these, however, I must put other things out of my mind and focus on the short-term process of completing the appropriate steps in the appropriate sequence to find out that $17 \times 24 = 408$.

Our long-term, System 1 memory operates on a fundamentally different basis than our shorter-term System 2 memory. As described by Kahneman, "System 1 runs automatically and System 2 is normally in a comfortable low-effort mode . . . System 2 is mobilized when a question arises for which System 1 does not offer an answer . . . Most of what you think and do originates in your System 1, but System 2 takes over when things get difficult" (pp. 24-25).

Much of the neuronal activity of the System 2 working memory occurs in the connections described in figure 8.4. The visual cortex and the auditory cortex connect with the prefrontal cortex through the associative cortex. Wernicke's area, discussed above as being involved in learning language and reading, is part of the associative cortex. As children get older, they experience increased myelination of the white matter connections between these areas. The more frequent the use of these connections, the greater the myelination of these connections. Klingberg (2013) reports that, based on studies his group has done, increased myelination in children is associated with improvements in working memory. Much in the same way that Yeatman reported less white-matter myelination in children who were weaker readers, Klingberg reports that in children, lower levels of myelination were also associated with lower working memory capacity.

If, as Kahneman suggests, most of what we do involves our System 1 memory, how does information get transferred from System 2 to System 1? The key to this transference process is the hippocampus, which is part of the temporal lobe. As an association passes through System 2 memory structures on a repeated basis, the hippocampus gradually transfers those associations to a different set of neurons. This new neuronal connection relies heavily on the prefrontal cortex to store them as long-term, System 1 memories. Eagleman describes this process as "rewir[ing] your own circuitry until it can accomplish the task with maximum efficiency. The task becomes burned into the machinery" (2011, p. 71).

Recall the study by Supekar described above, in which researchers identified in third-grade children an association between mathematical ability, the volume of the hippocampus, and the strength of the white-matter connections between the hippocampus and the prefrontal cortex. Recall also that Piaget suggested that children begin to develop mathematical ability when they enter the "concrete operational" phase of cognitive development, which begins at about age 7. As third-graders learn math, are they "rewiring" their brain circuitry in the way Eagleman suggests?

Research by Qin et al. (2014) addressed this question in a study of 28 children between the ages of 7 and 9, recruited from elementary schools in the San Francisco Bay Area. On two separate occasions separated by about 14 months, each child was asked to perform two age-appropriate mathematical calculations. One of these was done by having the child explain to the researcher how she or he solved the problem. The other was done while the child was undergoing an MRI scan on the brain. The questions the researchers were attempting to answer were (a) does the child's mathematical ability improve over this 14-month period, and (b) is there evidence that, over time, the children rely less on the counting strategies typical of System 2 working memory and more on rapid recall of answers from System 1 long-term memory? The answer was "yes" to both questions. The children's mathematical ability increased over the study period. For the first test, involving simple addition such as "4+1," the children relied more on the process of counting that uses working memory. By the second examination after 14 months, with slightly more complicated problems (e.g., 5 + 9), they relied less on counting and more on long-term memory to solve the problem.

The researchers then compared the results of the MRI scans at the two assessments. Consistent with the manner in which the children solved the problems verbally, while doing the problem in an MRI scanner, they used different parts of their brain to solve the problem. To solve the problem at the first assessment, they used principally the part of the brain involved in working memory. In solving the problems at the second assessment, they used less working memory, with greater activation of the hippocampus and its white-matter connections involved in long-term memory. From this the authors were able to conclude,

> We observed a shift from the use of counting to memory-based strategies in children over a 1.2-year interval, and this was associated with increased hippocampal engagement in problem solving . . . The increased hippocampal engagement is consistent with its known role in

learning and memory for encoding and retrieval of facts and events . . . Thus, our longitudinal findings suggest that the recruitment of hippocampal-dependent memory processes is important in the development of children's memory-based problem-solving strategies. (p. 6)

The authors then recruited and studied the mathematical ability of 20 adolescents between the ages of 14 and 17 and 20 young adults between the ages of 19 and 22. These older subjects were asked to solve more complex math problems. In doing so, the subjects relied heavily on long-term memory rather than the counting typical of short-term, working memory. In solving the problem while undergoing an MRI scan, these older subjects showed activity of the white-matter axonal connections involved in long-term System 1 memory without concurrent activation of the hippocampus. In these subjects, the work of the hippocampus in converting working memory to long-term memory was largely done. The adolescents and young adults had developed the myelinated axonal connections necessary to retrieve the memory required to solve the problem.

From these results the authors concluded that, at least in learning mathematics, "the hippocampus has a time-limited role in the early phase of knowledge acquisition . . . our findings suggest the hippocampal system is critical to children's early learning of arithmetic facts, the retrieval of which is largely dependent on the neocortex [long-term memory] in adults. Through further schooling and experience with mathematics, fact retrieval becomes increasingly independent of the hippocampal memory system during adolescence and adulthood" (Qin et al. 2014, p. 6). While the authors studied this process only in the developmental of mathematical ability, they suggested that the same processes may be involved in learning language and other academic abilities.

There certainly are ways to facilitate this process of transferring associations from the working memory to the long-term memory. Principal among these are repetition and practice. Landauer and Bjork (1978) describe their research on the optimal timing and spacing of this rehearsal process, which starts with immediate repetition and then spaces the repetitions at gradually increasing intervals.

For anyone who has learned to play a musical instrument as a child, this process may sound familiar. I certainly have seen it while watching my own son learn to play the piano. By the time he was a teenager, he had practiced his scales and chords enough times that he no longer had to invoke working memory to play them from the page of music. What did take practice, however, was learning to play them in a different sequence, with different tempo, different emphasis, and different fingering. One example comes particularly to mind— a piece by Aaron Copeland called *The Cat and the Mouse*. It involves some very complex transitions and sequences. He would practice a short section over and over and then leave it alone for a while. He'd come back to it in a day or two and do this again, only with increased facility. Gradually, a collection of short sequences began to blend into a wonderful piece of music, and gradually his eyes shifted from the notes on the page to the keys on the keyboard—he had memorized it. If you ever get a chance to hear this piece of music, you'll understand that it is not something one can play using System 2 working memory. One must let go of conscious control and let the music come spontaneously through the fingers to the piano. For his final recital, System 1 had taken over.

Klingberg suggests that the processes of learning to play a musical instrument are closely related to those of developing increased cognitive ability. He goes so far as to suggest that leaning a musical instrument may actually enhance cognitive ability, although he acknowledges that children who take music lessons often come from higher-income families with higher levels of parental education, so it is difficult to identify a clear causal relationship.

Emotional stress as another source of long-term memory

There is another type of long-term memory that does not follow this repetitive learning process. Often we can easily recall intensely emotional experiences, both positive and negative, even though they may have happened many years ago. These emotional experiences involve activation of the amygdala. As described in chapter 8, the amygdala plays a major role in sensing and managing emotion. When an unusually positive or negative emotion is experienced, the power of this experience can lead to neural connections through the hippocampus that create immediate, long-term memory. As part of this process, "stress hormones and stress-activated neurotransmitters enhance the consolidation of memory for emotionally arousing experiences through actions involving the amygdala. Such amygdala activation strengthens the storage of different kinds of information through the amygdala's widespread network of efferent projections to other brain regions" (Roozendaal et al. 2009, p. 423).

These memories, sometimes referred to as *flashbulb memories*, are "a vivid, enduring memory for how one learned about a surprising, shocking event" (Davidson et al. 2005, p. 915). In addition to remembering the emotion involved in the experience, one typically also remembers when and where the experience took place. Such memories are created through a process by which the amygdala sends neural impulses directly to the hippocampus and then through the hippocampus to the prefrontal cortex. When these memories are recalled, these connections are reactivated, including the perception of the emotion associated with the memory.

A secondary effect of this memory formation by joint activation of the amygdala and hippocampus is impairment of the usual functioning of the hippocampus in both working memory activities and the retrieval of other long-term memories. If the recall of these emotionally based memories occurs frequently, a significant consequence can be impairment of normal cognitive function. If they occur with sufficient force or severity they can result in mental illness such as post-traumatic stress disorder (PTSD) or other anxiety disorders. As described by Yehuda, "PTSD appears to represent a failure to recover from a nearly universal set of emotions and reactions and is typically manifested as distressing memories or nightmares related to the traumatic event, attempts to avoid reminders of the trauma, and a heightened state of physiological arousal" (2002, p. 113). These recurrent memories can substantially impede normal functioning and without treatment can lead to severe disability. Treatment usually involves a combination of medication and psychological counseling.

An interesting and potentially positive approach to reducing the effects of PTSD has been described by Schiller et al. (2009). Using a process called extinction training, they worked with people who had established fear memories by intentionally triggering those memories while simultaneously exposing the subject to new information unrelated to the previous trauma. For many of the subjects, the new memory overrode the old memory such that later triggering of the old memory no longer brought with it the powerful emotional response associated with activation of the amygdala. These results suggest that, as memories originating in the amygdala are transferred to the hippocampus and its connections with the prefrontal cortex, carefully introduced new memories could override the previous connection between the hippocampus and the amygdala, thus stripping the memory of much of its emotional content.

An additional impact of amygdala-related stress responses on the hippocampus has been identified, which we will discuss at greater length in chapter 10 as part of learning about the stress response. Repeated exposure to stress can cause atrophy of portions of the hippocampus, with resultant reductions in both working memory and long-term memory (McEwen 1999). Fortunately, it appears that "for the most part, these stress-induced changes in hippocampus and medial prefrontal cortex are reversible over time" (Roozendaal et al. 2009, p. 430). This is especially important to know, given that one of the most active periods for hippocampal growth, and as a consequence stress-related hippocampal impairment, is in early childhood.

Summary

As described above, we have come to understand cognition as knowing, attending, remembering, and reasoning. What we know starts out with the early perceptions of the environment and the development of language. It goes on to involve learning to read, learning to do math, and learning to manipulate abstract concepts. Piaget described this as a stepwise process that follows the various stages of neural development. Others see the process as more fluid, with less precise boundaries. However the process develops, our capacity to remember plays a central role.

We remember in two principal ways: with our long-term memory and with our shorter-term working memory. Kahneman (2011) refers to these as our System 1 memory and our System 2 memory. He emphasizes that much of our conscious awareness of day-to-day occurrences around us involves System 2. "When we think of ourselves, we identify with System 2, the conscious, reasoning self that has beliefs, makes choices, and decides what to think about and what to do" (p. 21). While System 2 is consciously at work, much of what we actually are doing is relying on the memories, associations, and learned behaviors stored in System 1. Especially in emergencies or unexpected situations, System 1 usually guides our reaction. While it's often System 1 that determines our moment-to-moment behaviors, System 2 still has the capability of taking over from System 1. As Kahneman describes, "most of what you (your System 2) think and do originates in your System 1, but System 2 takes over when things get difficult, and it normally has the last word" (2011, p. 25).

How we resolve this balance between thinking fast and thinking slow has a lot to do with how we see ourselves, our traits as seen by others, the goals we set for ourselves, and the very identity we adopt for ourselves. These aspects of cognition, motivation, and personality are central to our understanding of behavior. They are also aspects of development that can be powerfully affected by growing up in the context of social inequality and by experiencing abnormal levels of stress during childhood. The ways in which inequality and stress can affect behavior during childhood and adolescence and subsequent well-being are the issues I focus on in the following chapter.

REFERENCES

Adams, A. 2014. Stanford scientists discover a protein in nerves that determines which brain connections stay and which go, available at http://news.stanford.edu /news/2014/march/vision-brain-connections-033014 .html, accessed 5/1/14

American Psychological Association. Glossary of psycho logical terms, available at www.apa.org/research /action/glossary.aspx, accessed 5/1/14.

Clark, A., & Chalmers, D. 1998. The extended mind. Analysis 58(1): 7-19.

Davidson, P. S. R., Cook, S. P., Glisky, E. L., Verfaellie, M., & Rapcsak, S. Z. 2005. Source memory in the real world: A neuropsychological study of flashbulb memory. Journal of Clinical and Experimental Neuropsychology 27(7): 915-29.

Eagleman, D. 2011. Incognito: The Secret Lives of the Brain. New York: Vintage Books.

Fernald, A., Marchman, V. A., & Weisleder, A. 2013. SES differences in language processing skill and vocabulary are evident at 18 months. Developmental Science 16(2): 234-48.

Festa, N., Loftus, P. D., Cullen, M. R., & Mendoza, F. S. 2014. Disparities in early exposure to book sharing within immigrant families. Pediatrics 134(1): e162-68.

Hart, B., Risley, T. R. 1995. Meaningful Differences in the Everyday Experiences of Young American Children. Baltimore, MD: Brookes Publishing.

Kahneman, D. 2011. Thinking Fast and Thinking Slow. New York: Farrar, Straus and Giroux.

Klingberg, T. 2013. The Learning Brain: Memory and Brain Development in Children. New York: Oxford University Press.

Landauer, T. K., & Bjork, R. A. 1978. Optimum rehearsal patterns and name learning. In Gruneberg, M. M., Morris, P. E., & Sykes, R. N., eds. Practical Aspects of Memory, 625-32. London: Academic Press.

Lonigan, C. J., Burgess, S. R., & Anthony, J. L. 2000. Development of emergent literacy and early reading skills in preschool children: Evidence from a latent-variable longitudinal study. Developmental Psychology 36(5): 596-613.

McEwen, B. S. 1999. Stress and hippocampal plasticity. Annual Review of Neuroscience 22: 105-22.

Moon, C., Lagercrantz, H., & Kuhl, P. K. 2013. Language experienced in utero affects vowel perception after birth: A two-country study. Acta Paediatrica 102(2): 156-60.

Oxford English Dictionary, online edition, available at www.oed.com/, accessed 5/1/14.

Piaget, J. 1964. Development and learning. Journal of Research in Science Teaching 22(3): 176-86.

Qin, S., Cho, S., Chen, T., et al. 2014. Hippocampal-neocortical functional reorganization underlies children's cognitive development. Nature Neuroscience 17: 1263-69. doi: 10.1038/nn.3788.

Roozendaal, B., McEwen, B. S., & Chattarji, S. 2009. Stress, memory and the amygdala. Nature Reviews Neuroscience 10(6): 423-33.

Schiller, D., Monfils, M.-H., Raio, C. M., et al. 2009. Preventing the return of fear in humans using reconsolidation update mechanisms. Nature 63: 49-53.

Shonkoff, J. P., & Phillips, D. A., Eds. 2000. From Neurons to Neighborhoods: The Science of Early Childhood Development. National Academy Press, available at www.nap.edu/catalog.php?record_id =9824, accessed 5/12/14.

Shum, J., Hermes, D., Foster, B. L., et al. 2013. A brain area for visual numerals. Journal of Neuroscience 33(16): 6709-15.

Squire, L. R., & Zola, S. M. 1996. Structure and function of declarative and nondeclarative memory systems. Proceedings of the National Academy of Science USA 93(24): 13515-22.

Supekar, K., Swigart, A. G., Tenison, C., et al. 2013. Neural predictors of individual differences in response to math tutoring in primary-grade school children. Proceedings of the National Academy of Sciences USA 110(20): 8230-35.

Vygotsky, L. S. 1978. Mind in Society: The Development of Higher Psychological Processes. Cambridge, MA: President and Fellows of Harvard College.

Wandell, B. A., Rauschecker, A. M., & Yeatman, J. D. 2012. Learning to see words. Annual Review of Psychology 63: 31-53.

Weisleder, A., & Fernald, A. 2013. Talking to children matters: Early language experience strengthens processing and builds vocabulary. Psychological Science 24(11): 2143-52.

Yeatman, J. D., Dougherty, R. F., Ben-Shachar, M., & Wandell, B. A. 2012. Development of white matter and reading skills. Proceedings of the National Academy of Sciences USA 109(44): E3045-53.

Yehuda, R. 2002. Post-traumatic stress disorder. New England Journal of Medicine 346: 108-114.

chapter 10

Social Inequality, Childhood Experiences, and Behavior

The experience of inequality is directly associated with behaviors that impact well-being throughout the life course. Especially when economic inequality is combined with the social inequality of racial discrimination, a child growing up in these disadvantaged circumstances is at risk of developing strikingly different patterns of behavior than a child growing up in more advantaged circumstances. These behavioral differences will affect educational attainment as well as health-related behaviors as an adult and are a major contributor to existing disparities in life expectancy and quality of life. Having explored motivational development and the development of personality traits as well as cognitive development as it is related to neural development, we are now in a position to identify the specific mechanisms through which the early experience of inequality and the stressful experiences often associated with inequality can impact behavior and well-being.

Beginning in 2000, a series of reports by national research agencies began to address these issues. One of the first was a report of the Committee on Integrating the Science of Early Child Development, an interdisciplinary group established jointly by the National Research Council and the Institute of Medicine (IOM) of the National Academy of Sciences. The committee released its report in 2000 (Shonkoff and Phillips 2000). The charge to the committee was "to update scientific knowledge about the nature of early development and the role of early experiences, to disentangle such knowledge from erroneous popular beliefs or misunderstandings, and to discuss the implications of this knowledge base for early childhood policy, practice, professional development, and research" (p. 2).

In a later publication, the chair of the committee explained the assumptions on which the charge to the committee was based:

"First, that research on early childhood has been highly compartmentalized within discrete academic disciplines (e.g., psychology, neurobiology, and anthropology) . . . Second, that these diverse bodies of knowledge converge on a common core of shared concepts" (Shonkoff 2003, p. 70). From this, Shonkoff suggested, "The promising news is that the most important scientific breakthroughs in the future are likely to occur at the intersection of psychology, neurobiology, and molecular genetics" (p. 75).

By reviewing an extensive series of research reports, the committee identified a set of core concepts relating to early child development and offered a series of conclusions about how these concepts are related. Two of these conclusions have particular relevance for the issue of the impacts of inequality experienced during early childhood.

- "Early child development can be seriously compromised by social, regulatory, and emotional impairments."
- "Striking disparities in what children know and can do are evident well before they enter kindergarten. These differences are strongly associated with social and economic circumstances, and they are predictive of subsequent academic performance" (Shonkoff and Phillips 2000, p. 5).

In 2001, the IOM released another report, titled "Health and Behavior: The Interplay of Biological, Behavioral, and Societal Influences." In the report, a committee of scientists from a range of disciplines reviewed the available research addressing the mechanisms through which health and behavior are linked. One of the report's principal findings identified the link between the biological processes involved in early child development and the social context in which the child grows up.

A fundamental finding of the report is the importance of the interaction of psychosocial and biological processes in health and disease. Psychosocial factors influence health directly through biological mechanisms and indirectly through an array of behaviors. Social and psychological factors include socioeconomic status, social inequalities, social networks and support, work conditions, depression, anger, and hostility. (p. 16)

The report placed particular emphasis on how stressful experiences in early life can have potentially lifelong consequences. Referring to the role of stress-related hormones and allostatic load in affecting development, the authors underscored the ways in which "Changes in balance among neurotransmitters in the brain from the time of early development through adulthood to old age can influence behavioral responses to potentially stressful situations, can alter the interpretation of stimuli, and might be associated with anxiety and depression" (p. 4).

The report points to the consistent pattern found in the research literature that those who are poor and have a low level of education tend to engage in a range of behaviors that are detrimental to health. Given this broad pattern, the authors question the concept that behaviors principally reflect individual choice. Rather, the influence of social inequality, especially when experienced during the period of early neurological development, appears to lead to a range of unhealthy behaviors. It is the experience of inequality, rather than the characteristics unique to an individual, that lead to the broad pattern of behavior.

A subsequent IOM report released in 2006 followed up on these issues. One of the principal recommendations from that report was for developing new research efforts that focus on "the associations between health and interactions among social, behavioral, and genetic factors" and that "embraces the systems view and includes an examination of the interactive pathways through which these factors operate to affect health" (p. 3).

Since the publication of these reports, researchers from a range of disciplines have worked together to carry out the research called for by the reports. One of these groups, the National Scientific Council on the Developing Child, was formed in 2003, with Jack Shonkoff as its chair. In 2005 the group published a working paper titled "Excessive Stress Disrupts the Architecture of the Developing Brain." As the title suggests, the report focused on how stress experienced during infancy and early childhood can alter the neurological structure of the developing brain. Acknowledging that all children experience some form of stress as a normal part of development without suffering adverse consequences, the report differentiated three different types of stress.

- "*Positive stress* refers to moderate, short-lived stress responses, such as brief increases in heart rate or mild changes in the body's stress hormone levels. This kind of stress is a normal part of life, and learning to adjust to it is an essential feature of healthy development.
- "*Tolerable stress* refers to stress responses that have the potential to negatively affect the architecture of the developing brain but generally occur over limited time periods that allow for the brain to recover and thereby reverse potentially harmful effects.
- "*Toxic stress* refers to strong, frequent, or prolonged activation of the body's stress management system. Stressful events that are chronic, uncontrollable, and/or experienced without children having access to support from caring adults tend to provoke these types of toxic stress responses" (pp. 1–2)

Examples of positive stress include experiences such as meeting new people or getting an immunization. By overcoming these challenges, the child can develop in positive ways, gaining a sense that he or she can overcome these types of challenges in the future. Tolerable stress might be experienced as a result of an extremely frightening experience or a death in the family. So long as a child has loving, supportive adults who can help him or her through the experience, the stress need not result in harmful effects.

Toxic stress would come from experiences such as severe, ongoing abuse, either physical or emotional, especially if the abuse occurs during the periods of early childhood when the brain is developing its stress response systems. "Toxic stress during this early period can affect developing brain circuits and hormonal systems in a way that leads to poorly controlled stress response systems that will be overly reactive or slow to shut down when faced with threats throughout the lifespan" (p. 2).

Darlene Francis, a neuroscientist at the University of California, Berkeley, has focused her research on the ways in which social factors impact biological systems. In 2009 she published a paper describing how the expression of the genetic information contained in human DNA can be altered by factors in the physical or social environment in which a child grows up. Many people who learned a classical Mendelian approach to genetics understand the information contained in an individual's DNA and the resultant physiologic processes triggered by the nucleotide sequence in that DNA as fixed at conception and unchangeable, except through mutation. While the nucleotide sequence of DNA is largely fixed at conception, the way in which that genetic information is translated into physiologic processes (referred to as *gene expression*) can be affected by the biochemical environment in which the DNA exists. This includes the environment of the specific cell in which the DNA is situated, the environment of the organ system of which it is part, and the overall bodily environment as reflected in circulatory and neurological systems. While the information contained in the DNA sequence is referred to as the *genome*, the combination of factors in the surrounding environment that are capable of altering gene expression is referred to as the *epigenome*. As described by Francis, "The epigenome is innately plastic and can be programmed or reprogrammed by environmental experiences such as nutrition and stress. These epigenetic mechanisms provide the means through which social experiences can fundamentally and profoundly alter the regulation and expression of the genome without altering genotypes" (2009, p. S197). Francis points out that these epigenetic processes are extremely active during the early stages of development, both *in utero* and in infancy, when the child is growing most rapidly. Given that the social as well as the physical environment in which low-income and racial/ethnic minority children often grow up can be highly stressful, Francis suggests that these epigenetic mechanisms triggered by those environmental differences may contribute to health disparities later in life. "If we approach the question of racial/ethnic disparities in health from the perspective of developmental neurogenomics, we can begin to understand how different lived social experiences leave their epigenomic imprint on an organism" (p. S199).

Shonkoff et al. (2009) support this understanding that epigenetic changes triggered by stressful social or physical environments in early childhood are a major contributor to the continuing health disparities seen in adulthood, based on socioeconomic position and race/ethnicity. Considering data on adult disparities in conditions such as heart disease, stroke, diabetes, or cancer, they suggest that we not view existing disparities as solely the result of adult lifestyle and behavior. They suggest instead that "an extensive body of evidence linked adult chronic disease to processes and experiences occurring decades before, in some cases as early as intrauterine life, across a wide range of impairments" (p. 2253).

The American Academy of Pediatrics (AAP) created a task force to address the ways in which toxic stress experienced by children can lead to lifelong consequences on health. The group published its technical report in 2012 (Shonkoff et al.) The report recommends that pediatricians and other health care professionals address issues of child health from what they refer to as an "ecobiodevelopmental (EBD) framework." They describe how "Some of the most compelling new evidence for this proposed framework comes from the rapidly moving field of epigenetics, which investigates the molecular biological mechanisms (such as DNA methylation and histone acetylation) that affect gene expression without altering DNA sequence" (p. e234). They reiterate that this process begins in the early stages of development of the fetus *in utero* and continues in infancy, childhood, and beyond. They see child development as "driven by an ongoing, inextricable interaction between biology (as defined by genetic predispositions) and ecology (as defined by the social and physical environment)."

The report stresses that problems that develop during the educational process, such as lower levels of school readiness and lower academic attainment of children from disadvantaged backgrounds, can often be traced to these early developmental influences. Its authors suggest that stress experienced by young children be treated as a risk factor for subsequent unhealthy behaviors as adolescents and adults, much as cholesterol levels and blood pressure of younger adults are seen as risk factors for the development of cardiovascular problems later in life. They cite research showing that the brain architecture of school-aged children who earlier had experienced prolonged toxic stress demonstrates reduced hippocampal volume. As described in chapters 8 and 9, the hippocampus plays a major role in developing memory capacity as well as response patterns to environmental stimuli. As the authors describe, "Hence, altered brain architecture in response to toxic stress in early childhood could explain, at least in part, the strong association between early adverse experiences and subsequent problems in the development of linguistic, cognitive, and social-emotional skills, all of which are inextricably intertwined in the wiring of the developing brain" (Shonkoff et al. 2012, p. e236).

In addition to describing the reduced educational attainment and tendency toward adopting unhealthy behaviors that often accompany childhood exposure to toxic stress, the authors of the AAP report underscore the importance of the intergenerational transfer of these effects through an increased tendency of these individuals, when they reach late adolescence or early adulthood and have children of their own, to recreate an environment of toxic stress for their own children. The factors that contribute to higher stress, lower cognitive ability, more unhealthy behaviors, and reduced educational attainment are thus transferred across generations epigenetically, rather than genetically.

Based on the conclusions from this technical report, the American Academy of Pediatrics also published a policy statement targeting practicing pediatricians (AAP 2012). The key point the statement makes is that, despite the adverse impact of toxic stress on neural structure and hormonal stress regulation, the child's brain continues to exhibit *plasticity*—the ability to reshape itself in a more positive way in response to interventions that effectively target the origins of these early changes. The statement summarizes the findings of the technical report linking toxic stress experienced during childhood "to the subsequent development of unhealthy lifestyles (eg, substance abuse, poor eating and exercise habits), persistent socioeconomic inequalities (eg, school failure and financial hardship), and poor health (eg, diabetes and cardiovascular disease)" (p. e225).

The statement then goes on to suggest that "Given the extent to which costly health disparities in adults are rooted in these same unhealthy lifestyles and persistent inequalities, the reduction of toxic stress in young children ought to be a high priority for medicine as a whole and for pediatrics in particular." It also suggests that

it should be a primary role of pediatricians and other health professionals to identify the risk factors for and signs of toxic stress early in the life of children and to develop and test a series of interventions that will reverse the neurological and behavioral impacts of that stress. A principal focus of these interventions should be on helping the child's parents or other caregivers provide a consistently loving and supportive environment for the child, so that the long-term impacts of earlier stress can be minimized.

In 2014, the AAP held a national symposium to discuss the latest scientific and policy research and announced the creation of a new Center on Healthy, Resilient Children. As described in a press release, this new center "will be a national effort coordinated by the AAP and strategic partners to support healthy brain development and prevent toxic stress. In addition to prevention efforts to keep children healthy, the Center will focus on ways to help pediatricians and others identify children who have experienced adversity and toxic stress and ensure they have access to appropriate interventions and supports" (AAP 2014). It will be important to follow closely the research that comes from this new center and other research groups to learn what interventions have the best long-term outcomes on the behaviors and well-being of these vulnerable children.

Attention to addressing early childhood adversity from a prevention perspective is not confined to the United States. In 2009 the World Health Organization convened an international meeting, the title of which was Addressing Adverse Childhood Experiences To Improve Public Health. As a result of the discussion, participants agreed that the issue of adverse childhood experiences (ACE) should be seen as a major public health challenge. The meeting report concluded that "ACE work should be framed as an emerging field that highlights many massive prevention opportunities and raises questions about *how* ACE exposure can be reduced: the current challenge is not to fix the ACE problem, but to find out *how* to fix it" (p. 9).

Much of the terminology and many of the measurement instruments discussed at the World Health Organization meeting were based on work done by a collaborative project between the US Centers for Disease Control and Prevention and the Kaiser Permanente health care system in San Diego, California. In creating the Adverse Childhood Experiences (ACE) Study, the researchers developed a 10-question survey about a person's experiences during the first 18 years of life. Examples of questions on the survey, to be answered either "Yes" or "No," include:

- Did a parent or other adult in the household often or very often . . .
  - Swear at you, insult you, put you down, or humiliate you? *or*
  - Act in a way that made you afraid that you might be physically hurt?
- Did a parent or other adult in the household often or very often . . .
  - Push, grab, slap, or throw something at you? *or*
  - Ever hit you so hard that you had marks or were injured?
- Were your parents ever separated or divorced?

Responses to these questions yield an ACE Score ranging from 0 to 10. Using this score and the health data contained in the Kaiser Permanente electronic health record, researchers established associations between the ACE score and conditions such as smoking, alcohol use, depression, and suicide as well as many of the chronic medical conditions associated with the most common causes of premature death.

Socioeconomic inequality and early school readiness

In chapter 9, we saw how children growing up in families with lower socioeconomic status

(SES) entered school with reduced language capacity as well as lower reading ability. The work of Yeatman et al. described in chapter 9 identified reduced neurological development in the parts of the brain involved with reading for those children with reduced reading ability at age 7. Similarly, Noble et al. (2007) studied both performance assessment and brain structure of 150 first-graders drawn from diverse socioeconomic backgrounds. They found that it wasn't just language ability that was impaired in lower-SES children. Spatial cognition, memory, working memory, cognitive control, and reward processing were also reduced in children from lower-SES backgrounds, and these associations were continuous in nature, varying across all levels of SES.

As described in chapter 8, memory storage and retrieval as well as aspects of cognitive control are regulated largely by the hippocampus. Conditions that lead to atrophy in the hippocampus can also lead to reduced performance in declarative, episodic, spatial, and contextual memory (McEwen 1999). If, as Noble described, the memory and cognitive control of lower-SES children is reduced relative to their higher-SES classmates, this raises the question of whether there might be an association between poverty, stress, and the development of the hippocampus. This is the question Luby et al. (2013) addressed in a study of 145 children between the ages of 6 and 12. The children were initially part of a longitudinal study of preschool children between the ages of 3 and 6. As part of that study children were assessed for having experienced stressful life events, the quality of the care provided by the parent or other caregiver, and the families' socioeconomic characteristics such as income and parental education. Family income was measured as the ratio of actual income to financial need as indicated by the federal poverty level based on family size.

Between ages 6 and 12, the researchers administered an MRI brain scan to evaluate each child's brain structure, with particular atten-

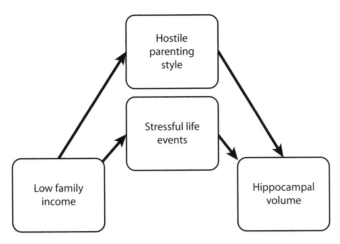

FIGURE 10.1. The Association between Family Income, Adverse Early Childhood Experiences, and Hippocampal Volume. From Luby et al. 2013.

tion paid to the volume of the hippocampus within the brain as well as to the volume of cortical gray matter and white matter in other parts of the brain. They found a significant association between income and the volume of the hippocampus, cortical gray matter, and cortical white matter. Children from lower-income families, typically having parents with lower levels of education, consistently had reduced neural capacity in all these areas.

The researchers then studied whether they would still find this association between family income and hippocampal volume if they also entered into the analysis measures of the stressful life events experienced by the child before entering school and of the level of hostile parenting style exhibited by the parents. Their results are shown in figure 10.1.

After taking into account separate measures of parenting style and having experienced stressful life events, there was no longer a direct association between family income and hippocampal volume. The authors did find that lower family income was associated both with more frequent occurrence of hostile parenting practices on the part of the child's parents and with experiencing stressful life events more fre-

quently as a young child. They also found that each of these measures—hostile parenting and stressful life events—was independently associated with reduced hippocampal volume. However, in the model that included all three variables, family income no longer showed an association with hippocampal volume. These results suggest that it is not low family income per se that leads to reduced hippocampal volume in children. Rather, it is the occurrence of hostile parenting and stressful life events that reduces hippocampal volume and the cognitive capacity that goes along with it. Parents in low-income families, who are likely to have lower levels of educational attainment themselves, are more likely to engage in hostile parenting toward their young children and more likely to have a home environment that young children experience as highly stressful. In discussing these results, the authors commented, "The key role of caregiver nurturance in hippocampal development and its relationship to adaptive stress responses has been well established in animal studies . . . Thus, the current findings add to and extend the literature underscoring the critical role of nurturance for childhood well-being" (Luby et al. 2013, p. 1141).

The journal that published this study by Luby et al. also published an editorial comment on the results. In it, Nelson underscored the significance of the implications of this research:

> Whether we adopt the term *developmental programming* or *biological embedding*, the construct remains the same: early experience weaves its way into the neural and biological infrastructure of the child in such a way as to impact developmental trajectories and outcomes . . . If we wish to protect our children's brains, we must work hard to protect their young minds. Exposure to early life adversity should be considered no less toxic than exposure to lead, alcohol, or cocaine, and, as such, it merits similar attention from public health authorities. (2013, p. 1098)

If children from socioeconomically disadvantaged families are at higher risk of experiencing hostile parenting and other forms of stress, how are the associated reductions in hippocampal and cortical brain functioning likely to show up once the child enters school? Boyce et al. (2012) addressed this question in a study of 338 5-year-old kindergarteners recruited from public schools in Berkeley, California. Consistent with the demographics of Berkeley, the children were from a diverse range of families, including low-income and high-income, with parents with less than a high school education to parents with a graduate or professional degree. The researchers observed the children's interactions in the classroom and gathered information from the teachers about their perceptions of the children's level of adaptability, classroom functioning, and emotional state. From these data the researchers developed a series of multi-item measures. They also had a separate measure of academic competence. They found that children from lower-SES families showed more evidence of depression and more frequent inattention as well as exhibiting less "prosocial behavior" and having weaker

peer relationships. The lower-SES children, as we might now expect, were also less academically competent than their higher-SES peers.

The researchers also found one additional outcome of interest. They noted that the children tended to establish status relationships among themselves, with certain children taking on dominant social roles while interacting with classmates and others taking on subordinate roles. They found that neither gender nor SES seemed to play a role in which children would assume dominant social roles and which would become subordinate. However, of children in a subordinate position, those from lower-SES families seemed to respond more negatively, with lower levels of prosocial behavior with peers. From these observations, the authors concluded that "socioeconomic gradients in health and development are the products of more than simply differences in access to money, material goods, medical care, or nutrition. Rather, the evidence implies that even the stratification of young children's peer groups is implicated in the diverging trajectories of lifelong health" (Boyce et al. 2012, p. 17171).

Another research group assessed the relationship between the SES context in which a child grows up and her or his level of cognitive development in kindergarten (Noble et al. 2005) and first grade (Noble et al. 2007). They evaluated 60 kindergarten children in Philadelphia, half from low-SES families and half from middle-SES families, administering standardized tests of visual, spatial, memory, language, and executive cognitive functioning. They found lower average cognitive ability in the lower-SES children in all five areas, particularly in language and executive function.

In the second study, first-grade children were selected from nine different schools in New York City that represented a range of socioeconomic backgrounds. Researchers evaluated the children's language, spatial cognition, memory (both long-term and working memory), cognitive control, and reward processing systems.

They found that "language, spatial cognition, memory, and some but not all executive abilities vary continuously with SES" (Noble et al. 2007, p. 476).

While the hippocampus regulates memory and cognitive function, the amygdala, which is located adjacent to the hippocampus, plays a major role in regulating emotions and response to stress. Overactivity of the amygdala on a sustained basis can impede hippocampal function. Based on the research of Luby and others, we have seen evidence that toxic levels of stress experienced during early childhood, often associated with lower-SES family environments, is associated with impaired development of the hippocampus. Will toxic levels of stress during early childhood also affect the size and activity of the amygdala, and will children with increased amygdala activity exhibit higher levels of anxiety? Qin et al. reviewed the research in this area, much of which has been done in laboratory animals, and concluded that "Early life stress and anxiety have been linked to enlarged amygdala ... resulting from interplay of prolonged over-activity of stress-sensitive hormones and experience-dependent plasticity in the developing animal brain" (2014, p. 892)

Qin's research team performed MRI scans of the brains of 76 children between the ages of 7 and 9. The sample size and demographics of the study group were not sufficient to make comparisons based on family SES or the frequency of stressful childhood experiences. Rather, the researchers assessed the level of anxiety exhibited by each child, based on parental reports using standardized assessment instruments. They then compared the size of the amygdala with the level of anxiety exhibited by each child and found a significant association, with those children exhibiting greater levels of anxiety also tending to have greater amygdala volume. Commenting on the implications of this association for later child health and development, the authors concluded that "amygdala hyperconnectivity in anxious children has a

neuroanatomical profile similar to those seen in adults with high anxiety ... Interaction between stress exposure and altered amygdala circuitry may exacerbate vulnerability toward anxiety disorders" (Qin et al. 2014, p. 898).

Shonkoff (2012) emphasizes the time of entry into school as having special significance for children for two reasons. First, a child's ability to focus attention, manage feelings and emotions, control impulses, learn and follow rules, and adapt to changing circumstances are essential to subsequent academic success. In the eyes of many teachers, these early capacities are more important than a child's knowledge of numbers and letters. Second, the years leading up to school entry are a time of some of the most rapid changes in brain structure in terms of developing the capacity for this type of "executive function," as Shonkoff describes these abilities. "The acquisition of executive function and self-regulatory skills corresponds closely to the extended development of the prefrontal cortex, which begins in early infancy and continues into the early adult years. Because these neural circuits have extensive interconnections with deeper brain structures that control responses to threat and stress, maturing executive functioning both influences, and is affected by, a young child's management of strong emotions" (p. 17302).

We thus can expect many children from disadvantaged socioeconomic backgrounds, especially those who experience high levels of stress at home during early childhood, to have a disruption in the structure of the amygdala and the hippocampus such that their executive function may be impaired and the level of anxiety they experience will increase in a new environment such as school. A study by Kamp Dush et al. (2013) suggested that these children may also experience worse physical health as a result of the "chaos" they experience in the home environment.

The Center on the Developing Child at Harvard University (2011) has reviewed current scientific knowledge of the development of and key components of executive function in young children. Consistent with Shonkoff's perspective, the center defines executive function in children as "a group of skills that helps us to focus on multiple streams of information at the same time, monitor errors, make decisions in light of available information, revise plans as necessary, and resist the urge to let frustration lead to hasty actions" (p. 1). These executive function capacities are necessary not only to adapt successfully to the school environment but also to engage successfully in the process of learning to read and acquiring basic mathematical skills. "Scientists who study executive function skills refer to them as the biological foundation for school readiness. They argue that strong working memory, cognitive self-control, and attentional skills provide the basis upon which children's abilities to learn to read, write, and do math can be built" (p. 4).

The center's report identifies three key components of executive function.

- Working memory—In chapter 9 we differentiated working memory from long-term memory. Working memory addresses currently available information and manipulates it in ways that allow us to solve new problems, whether they are mathematical or behavioral.
- Inhibitory control—In chapter 6 we discussed the factors that contribute to a child's motivation to respond to circumstances in a particular way. Recall the example of the 4-year old children in the Mischel study deciding whether to wait for two marshmallows or to ring the bell now and take one marshmallow. In circumstances such as these, children are able to use their thought process and conscious control mechanisms to avoid distractions and to counterbalance feelings of wanting to act impulsively.

- Cognitive or mental flexibility—These capacities enable children to adapt to rapidly changing circumstances and to adjust behavior accordingly. Talking one-on-one with a classmate in school will be different from talking with a teacher or with a group of students. Well-adjusted children will respond somewhat differently in each of these settings.

As described in the report, teachers will often pay principal attention to a child's level of executive function in determining school readiness. They know that both successful learning and successful social interaction depend on these different aspects of executive function. The report cites research by Welsh et al. (2010) showing that children from low-income families who exhibit problems in executive function upon entering Head Start preschool showed lower increases in reading and math preparation during preschool than those with greater executive function, even after controlling for the child's reading and math ability upon entering preschool.

While the development of executive function continues throughout childhood and into adolescence, the report identifies the period between the ages of about 18 months and 5 years as the most rapid in this developmental process. This is precisely the time period during which children from disadvantaged socioeconomic circumstances and stressful family environments will be impacted the most in terms of their subsequent success in school. In summarizing its analysis, the report concludes, "Mounting evidence is revealing the roles played by community, school, and family contexts, as well as socioeconomic status, in the development of executive function skills. Children from lower (versus higher) socioeconomic backgrounds show poorer performance on tests of working memory, cognitive flexibility, and inhibition, as well as electrophysiological evidence of altered prefrontal functioning between ages 7 to 12" (p. 7).

Noble et al. (2005) studied public school children in Philadelphia, 30 from middle-SES families and 30 from lower-SES families. They compared the children on a range of neurocognitive capacities. Consistent with the finding of the previous study, they also found that family SES was strongly associated with two of these capacities, language and executive function, with lower-SES children in kindergarten demonstrating lower capacities in both.

What are the implications for a child entering kindergarten who has grown up in stressful or disadvantaged circumstances and who, as a consequence, has the reduced hippocampal volume described above by Luby et al. (2013), with consequent delayed development of executive functioning? Portilla et al. (2014) studied 338 5-year old children in the San Francisco Bay Area, drawn from diverse SES and racial/ethnic backgrounds. Shortly after the children first entered kindergarten, researchers assessed each child using standardized survey instruments and information provided by the parents and

teacher. They measured two principal behaviors of the children while they were in kindergarten: inattention and impulsivity, and school engagement. Separately, they asked the teacher of each child to evaluate their perception of the teacher-child relationship and whether the teacher viewed the relationship with that child as conflictual.

They followed the children throughout kindergarten in order to measure these factors at both the beginning of kindergarten and the end of kindergarten. They then re-evaluated each child at the end of first grade to measure that child's academic competence at that time as well as the quality of the teacher-child relationship as reported by the first grade teacher. Finally, they asked if the behaviors observed at the beginning of the kindergarten year were associated with subsequent behaviors, with the quality of the teacher-child relationship, and with academic competence in first grade. The results of the study are shown in figure 10.2.

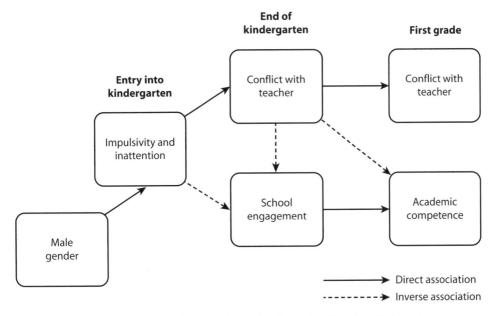

FIGURE 10.2. Association between Executive Control on Entering Kindergarten and Learning Outcomes. From Portilla et al. 2014.

The first thing to notice is that, upon entry to kindergarten, boys on average exhibited more impulsivity and inattention than girls. Regardless of gender, those children who earlier had shown impulsivity and inattention were, by the end of kindergarten, viewed by the teacher as more conflictual. Two factors independently predicted the level of school engagement at the end of kindergarten: having demonstrated impulsivity and inattention at the beginning of kindergarten and being seen by the teacher as more conflictual.

Not surprisingly, those students who demonstrated less engagement in school during kindergarten were also found to be less academically competent in first grade. In addition, those children whose relationship with the teacher was seen by the teacher as conflictual also showed lower academic competence in first grade. In an important and yet worrisome finding, those children seen as conflictual by the kindergarten teacher were also more likely to be seen as conflictual by the first-grade teacher. The extent to which the kindergarten teacher had conveyed information directly to the first-grade teacher about a child's tendency to be conflictual is not known.

It seems that children from disadvantaged social backgrounds who demonstrate weak executive functioning upon entering kindergarten are at risk of being labeled as problem children by the kindergarten teacher. This label may then stay with the child as she or he progresses into higher grades. In reporting these findings, Portilla's team suggests that "The strong effect of inattention and impulsive behaviors on teacher-child relationship quality began at the transition into elementary school, pointing to a need for strategies to help young children develop stronger self-regulatory skills in preschool and earlier" (2014, p. 1927).

Acknowledging and underscoring the importance for young children of developing executive control and the capacity to self-regulate, the Administration for Families and Children of the US Department of Health and Human Services commissioned a series of reports on the topic from the Center for Child and Social Policy at Duke University. The first of these reports, titled *Self-Regulation and Toxic Stress: Foundations for Understanding Self-Regulation from an Applied Developmental Perspective*, was published in 2015 (Murray et al.). The authors of the report reviewed an extensive literature addressing a range of topics related to the development of self-regulation by children and identified seven core principles that summarize current understanding of the development of self-regulation.

1. Self-regulation serves as the foundation for lifelong functioning across a wide range of domains, from mental health and emotional wellbeing to academic achievement, physical health, and socioeconomic success. It has also proven responsive to intervention, making it a powerful target for change.
2. Self-regulation is defined from an applied perspective as the act of managing cognition and emotion to enable goal-directed actions such as organizing behavior, controlling impulses, and solving problems constructively.
3. Self-regulation enactment is influenced by a combination of individual and external factors including biology, skills, motivation, caregiver support, and environmental context.
4. Self-regulation can be strengthened and taught like literacy, with focused attention, support, and practice opportunities provided across contexts.
5. Development of self-regulation is dependent on "co-regulation" provided by parents or other care-giving adults through warm and responsive interactions . . .
6. Self-regulation can be disrupted by prolonged or pronounced stress and adversity including poverty and trauma experiences . . . Stress that overwhelms children's skills or support

can create toxic effects that negatively impact development and produce long-term changes in neurobiology.

7. There are two clear developmental periods where self-regulation skills increase dramatically due to underlying neurobiological changes—early childhood and adolescence—suggesting particular opportunities for intervention. (Murray et al. 2015, p. 3)

These principles bring together many of the issues we have covered in previous chapters as well as earlier in this chapter. As a natural part of the early developmental process, children learn, to various degrees, the cognitive and emotional skills that allow them to respond to environmental stimuli through their behavior. In much the same way that learning to read involves a succession of sensory experiences that guide the development of neural structures linking together various specialized cortical areas of the brain, learning to self-regulate involves an analogous process. As principle six above describes, however, this process "can be disrupted by prolonged or pronounced stress and adversity including poverty and trauma experiences." Those children who experience this disruption are at increased risk of entering school with a combination of weak self-regulation and impaired cognitive development. The adverse impact of these disadvantages on subsequent engagement in school and academic ability make these children at greater risk of developing unhealthy behavioral patterns as adolescents that can affect subsequent well-being as an adult. As Murray et al. describe, "Indeed, self-regulation has been identified as the foundation for lifelong physical and mental health" (p. 4).

It is crucial that we fully appreciate both the seriousness of these risks and the fact that they are not necessarily permanent. As Murray et al. go on to describe, "just as a child who struggles with literacy for any number of reasons may later become literate when provided with effec-

tive instruction in a supportive environment, we believe that children who have early self-regulation difficulties are capable of acquiring these skills at later ages" (p. 13). Given what Murray et al. describe as "co-regulation"—the experience of supportive interactions over time with a sensitive and caring adult such as a teacher or counselor—a child has the potential to catch up on self-regulatory capacity by the time he or she is an adolescent, in much the same way that a slow reader can improve his or her reading through practice and support.

In 2014, *New York Times* columnist David Brooks published an op-ed commentary titled "The Character Factory." Brooks cited research showing that "measures of drive and self-control influence academic achievement roughly as much as cognitive skills." A principal point he made in his commentary was that government-supported programs for early childhood education need to focus as much on the development of character as on the development of specific academic skills. "Recent research has also shown that there are very different levels of self-control up and down the income scale. Poorer children grow up with more stress and more disruption, and these disadvantages produce effects on the brain . . . But these effects are reversible with the proper experiences."

In 2014, Neil Halfon from the Center for Healthier Children, Families, and Community at the UCLA School of Medicine published an editorial in *JAMA* addressing the "Socioeconomic Influences on Child Health." In it, he argued that

new research on the development of 'executive function' documents how the capacity for impulse control, persistence, and focused attention formed in the early years is predictive of health, behavioral, and educational outcomes, and is sensitive to the poverty-associated effects of stress. In other words, poverty impedes the development of the neurobiological mechanisms that enable individuals to make appropriate choices and resist the temptations to overeat, smoke, drink excessively, and use drugs, thereby placing children in this environment at increased risk for a wide range of health problems throughout their lives. (Halfon 2014, p. 916)

The neurological, cognitive, and behavioral disadvantages experienced by young children from disadvantaged backgrounds need not be seen as irreversible. Increased focus on supporting parents and preschool as well as school programs that develop children's executive function as well as reading and math skills can help prevent many of the behavioral consequences of early disadvantage that begin to show up in adolescence.

The impact of social disadvantage on adolescent development

Elementary school-age children demonstrate in a number of ways the adverse impacts of early childhood stress. As we have described, they are at risk of worse health status, higher levels of anxiety, lower levels of executive function, and lower educational attainment. While these effects may be open to change through well designed interventions, without such interventions we can expect children to continue to experience these outcomes as adolescents.

Recent research has documented these effects in adolescence in a number of ways. Dowd et al. (2014) analyzed data from the National Longitudinal Study of Adolescent Health, a nationally representative sample of adolescents. They found a strong association between having come from a lower-SES family and two measures of stress: perceived stress level and the frequency of experiencing stressful life events during adolescence. They found that, at comparable income levels, black adolescents experienced more stress during adolescence than white adolescents.

Using the same data set, Bauldry et al. (2012) explored the association between stressful

events during childhood and self-rated health (SRH) during adolescence and young adulthood. As the authors describe, "Background characteristics (parental education, income, and family structure), parental health conditions (asthma, diabetes, obesity, migraines), and early health challenges (physical abuse, presence of a disability, and parental alcoholism and smoking) predict SRH from adolescence to young adulthood" (p. 1311). In their analysis, the authors note that the health-related behaviors the subjects adopted during adolescence, such as smoking, obesity, and alcohol use, had a substantial impact on their SRH during adolescence and into young adulthood.

Machado-de-Sousa et al. (2014), in a study of students entering university in Brazil, used MRI scans to see whether those students exhibiting higher levels of anxiety would have any change in the structure of their amygdala. Compared to those students not exhibiting evidence of anxiety, those with personal or social anxiety had greater volume of the amygdala. While the study did not include subjects for whom there was a record of stress exposure during childhood, these results nonetheless suggest that the adverse health outcomes experienced by adolescents who had experienced toxic stress as young children are likely associated with persistent structural changes in the amygdala and a high level of hormonal and neural response in potentially stressful situations.

Blair et al. (2014) published a review article about factors that affect conduct problems in children and adolescents. As they describe, "The term 'conduct problems' refers to a pattern of repetitive rule-breaking behavior, aggression, and disregard for others" (p. 2207). They go into some depth describing the neurological structures and functions associated with conduct problems and conclude that "environmental risks confer a predisposition to conduct problems through effects on neurocognitive function. Risk factors with a postnatal effect include low levels of parental monitoring, exposure to violence, and harsh and inconsistent discipline, as well as circumstances, such as poverty, in which the other risk factors tend to coalesce" (p. 2213).

Given these effects of childhood stress on adolescents and evidence that those having experienced high levels of stress are more likely to adopt unhealthy behaviors as adolescents, it is important to understand how these behaviors are initially adopted. In chapter 4 I described the many ways that, as children grow into adolescence, social networks play an increasingly significant role in influencing both perceptions and behavior. As those networks expand to include school peers, and as the adolescent begins to separate his or her identity from that of parents, peer expectations and behaviors began to exert greater influence. Particularly as one moves into high school, peer groups often differentiate into those who experience academic success and those with lower academic success. Those students who, during early adolescence, develop a greater sense of what Pachucki et al. (2015) refer to as "school connectedness"—feeling close to people at school, feeling happy to be at school, feeling themselves to be part of the school, and feeling as though they are treated fairly by teachers—exhibit greater levels of self-esteem on a standardized psychological assessment. Self-esteem can be a key component of a feeling of self-efficacy. Those with greater academic success and a greater sense of self-efficacy are likely to adopt a Future perspective, as described in chapter 6. Those peers with lower academic success will, by contrast, feel more disconnected from school and may begin to adapt more risky behaviors, consistent with the Zimbardo's Present-Fatalistic and Present-Hedonistic time perspectives.

Those adolescents who adopt a present-hedonistic perspective will focus less on the long-term effects of their behavior and more on the immediate enjoyment and pleasure they derive from a behavior. A principal example of

this type of behavior among adolescents is alcohol use. Fujimoto and Valente (2015) assessed the impact of peer relationships in a study of 1707 high school students in California, predominantly from low-income Hispanic families. They found that a principal predictor of whether a student had begun to drink alcohol was having a close friend who had also begun to drink alcohol. Thus, choosing to associate with others who drink alcohol appears to increase the likelihood that an adolescent himself or herself will also start to drink.

While alcohol is an important contributor to adult health disparities, as described in chapter 2, cigarette smoking, diet, and exercise each has a substantially more profound impact on adult well-being and premature death than alcohol use alone. We also saw consistent evidence that those with lower levels of education were, as adults, more likely to smoke and to be obese. Hanson and Chen (2007) reviewed research on the impact of having grown up in a low-SES family on health behaviors in adolescence. They found consistent evidence that those adolescents who grew up in low-SES circumstances were more likely to smoke, to have a poor diet, and to exercise less. In their review, they did not find consistent evidence that low SES was associated with greater alcohol use by adolescents. Nor did they find evidence of consistent racial or ethnic differences in these behaviors, after SES had been taken into account.

Hanson and Chen noted that those growing up in a low-SES household were likely also to have parents with low educational attainment. Since those adults with low educational attainment are also more likely to smoke, they postulated that children in low-SES families would be more likely to observe their own parents smoking and might therefore model their own behavior as adolescents on their parents as well as their peers. As described by the authors, "Taken together, parent modeling and attitudes, as well as the experience of stress and negative life events, may lead low SES teens to be more likely to try cigarettes than high SES teens" (p. 277).

Poonawalla et al. (2014) also looked at the association of family SES and adolescent behaviors, focusing on smoking and alcohol use. Their study involved 1,356 mostly white subjects who had been followed from birth through 15 years of age. They looked both at overall family SES, measured as being above or below 200 percent of the federal poverty line, and at change in family income between the time the child was 1 month old and 15 years old. As with the earlier study, they found that children in lower-income families both at birth and as adolescents were more likely to smoke at age 15. They again noted that the rate of maternal smoking was also higher in the lower-income families, providing a modeling effect. While low income itself was not associated with alcohol use at 15, a downward income trajectory over that time period, suggesting more stressful family circumstances due to reduced SES, was associated with the rate of alcohol use at age 15.

Boynton-Jarrett et al. (2013) reported on their research that described the cumulative effects of turbulence experienced during childhood and adolescence and several key outcomes during adolescence: health risk behavior, mental health, and completion of high school. Using representative national data from a longitudinal study of children aged 12–14, they asked how socioeconomic factors such as parents' age, education, and occupation, family income, and family structure and processes were associated with these adolescent behaviors. Consistent with the discussions above, they found that those adolescents coming from more turbulent home backgrounds were more likely to smoke, more likely to be sexually active, more likely to experience mental health problems, somewhat more likely to belong to a gang, and less likely to graduate from high school. Given the importance high school graduation plays in affecting lifelong health behaviors, we clearly see the roots of reduced adult well-being being in place well before a child moves into adulthood.

The added impact of minority race

So far our discussion of socioeconomic disadvantage has focused primarily on parental income and education, home environment, social environment, and the influence of positive school connectedness. Racial discrimination, principally as experienced by African Americans, is another form of social disadvantage that can have profound impacts on adolescent behaviors. Bogart et al. (2013) evaluated data on about 5,000 fifth-grade students from three different communities, with roughly equal numbers of white, black, and Latino students. They asked these children whether they had been treated badly because of their race or ethnicity or because of the color of their skin. They compared those children who answered yes to either of these questions to those who answered no to both. They then compared the children on scales of physical aggression, verbal aggression, and delinquent behavior, as reported by the children themselves. They found that, after controlling for socioeconomic differences, both black and Latino students who had experienced discrimination were more likely than those who had not to exhibit these problem behaviors. Overall, black students exhibited more problem behaviors than white students, with about half of that difference associated with the high rate of having experienced discrimination among the black students. Interestingly, after controlling for socioeconomic factors, the overall rate of problem behaviors among the Latino students was lower than among the white students.

Priest et al. (2013) reviewed an extensive series of research articles about the impact of having experienced racial discrimination on the well-being of those age 12–18. They summarized the results of their review as "provid[ing] compelling evidence for acknowledging and addressing racial discrimination as a key determinant of health for children and young people by documenting strong and consistent relationships between reported racial discrimination and a range of detrimental health outcomes across various age groups, racial/ethnic backgrounds and settings" (p. 122). The types of outcomes they assessed included mental health (anxiety, depression, and psychological distress) and reduced self-esteem or sense of self-worth. While these outcomes were found in a range of minority racial or ethnic groups, one finding in particular applied principally to black youth: a strong association between having experienced racial discrimination and engaging in delinquent behaviors.

Sanders-Phillips et al. (2009) emphasized the importance of a diminished sense of control over life as a worrisome outcome of the experience of racial discrimination during childhood. In black families especially, that perceived loss of control can affect mothers as well as their children. A mother who perceives less self-efficacy in being able to provide her child with a supportive home environment may develop lower parenting skills, resulting in a weaker parent-child relationship. That loss of parental nurturing and support can reduce the child's own sense of self-efficacy, with that loss "associated with risk behaviors such as drug use, aggression, and sexual risk-taking" (p. S180).

Sanders-Phillips goes on to acknowledge a potentially more worrisome outcome of the experience of racial discrimination during childhood, described as anomie. "Anomie, which is characterized by feelings of hopelessness and perceptions of little control over life outcomes (i.e., decreased self-efficacy), develops when children perceive contradictions between opportunities in the larger society and the conditions and lack of opportunity in their own lives. Racial discrimination increases anomie by reinforcing perceptions of inequality and limiting options for achieving life goals" (p. S178). As children and adolescents view the impacts of

racial discrimination on those close to them, they not only can develop a sense of hopelessness but also can develop a deep sense of distrust of others, especially those in higher-SES positions who are not black.

This continuing evidence of black youth in the United States experiencing racial discrimination brings up a related question: the direct impact of experiencing racial discrimination on physiological health, in particular cardiovascular health. In chapter 8 we discussed the ways in which a chronically elevated allostatic load— the level of stressor hormones circulating in the body—is often the result of chronic or recurrent environmental stressors perceived by the stress regulatory mechanism of the brain and autonomic nervous system. If that stress is severe and persists over time, the chronic elevation in the stress response hormones, principally cortisol, epinephrine, and norepinephrine, can begin to cause injury to the cells lining the blood circulatory system, principally the arteries and smaller arterioles (McEwen 1998, Seeman et al. 2010).

Heffernan et al. (2008) studied the arterial system in 25 young (average age of 23), healthy black men and compared the results with those from 30 white men of the same age and health status. One of the tests they performed was an ultrasound analysis of the carotid artery, the artery that can be felt in the side of the neck. They found that, compared to the white men, the carotid arteries in the young black men were, on average, stiffer and had a thicker wall, suggesting scarring of the lining of the artery such as that associated with chronically elevated allostatic load.

Will black adolescents, many of whom have experienced repeated racial discrimination while growing up, also exhibit thicker and stiffer arteries than comparable white adolescents? Thurston and Matthews (2009) also used ultrasound analysis to measure the stiffness and wall thickness of the carotid artery in 81 black and 78 white adolescents with a mean age of 17.8 years.

They found that both lower SES and black race were associated with thicker and stiffer arteries, with the strongest effect shown for low-SES black youth. It thus appears that, especially for black youth, experiencing racial discrimination during childhood and adolescence will compound the adverse physiologic impacts of growing up in lower-SES circumstances.

Adolescent educational attainment as reflecting parents' educational attainment

We have known for some time that one of the strongest predictors of an adolescent's educational attainment is the level of education his or her parents were able to attain. A 2001 federal report from the National Center for Education Statistics showed that 82 percent of students whose parents had at least a bachelor's degree went to college immediately after finishing high school, while 36 percent of students whose parents had not completed high school went to college after high school. In certain high-poverty communities, the rates were even lower. A 25-year study of children growing up in Baltimore conducted by Johns Hopkins University sociologist Karl Alexander (Rosen 2014) showed that only 4 percent of children growing up in low-income families had completed a bachelor's degree by age 28, as compared to 45 percent of children in Baltimore from higher-income families. Much of this failure to attain a college education reflects the extremely high rates of dropping out of high school of low-income students and students in certain racial or ethnic minority groups. Of 16-to-24-year-olds nationally from families in the lowest quartile of income, approximately 12 percent had dropped out of high school before completion. For blacks or Hispanics in this age range, 9 percent and 14 percent, respectively, had not completed high school (National Center for Education Statistics 2014).

Why do the children of parents with a low level of educational attainment tend also to attain less education themselves? Given the powerful influence of educational attainment on lifelong well-being, this question is central to our understanding of the ways in which social disadvantage affects the behaviors of adolescents. Davis-Kean (2005) examined cross-sectional data on a nationally representative sample that included 868 children between the ages of 8 and 12. The sample was evenly split between white and black children in families with a range of incomes. She explored the associations between the parents' level of education and the child's score on a standardized achievement test. While there was an association between parents' educational level and the child's score on the achievement test, it was largely an indirect relationship. It turned out that parents' education was associated with several dynamics of the home environment, including the expectations the parents expressed for their child's subsequent educational attainment and the extent to which the child was reading books on a regular basis. After taking these factors into account, the direct association between parents' education and children's achievement was substantially diminished.

Commenting on these and similar results, Eccles and Davis-Kean (2005) point out that the quality of the neighborhood environment will also vary in association with parents' level of education and that environment can in turn affect the child's educational attainment. In their summary of their research, however, they underscore the conclusion that "Both existing studies and the research summarized in this paper document the link between various parental characteristics, beliefs and behaviors and their children's educational attainments. We have shown that the relation of parents' education to their children's academic achievement and motivation is mediated by quite specific beliefs and behaviors" (p. 201).

This conclusion—that it is the impact of parental education on parental and child beliefs and attitudes that is largely responsible for the association between parental and child educational attainment—is supported by the research of Dubow et al. (2009), referenced earlier in chapter 1. They used data from a longitudinal study of 856 children in a semirural area of New York State who were in the third grade in 1960. The study recontacted the subjects at ages 19, 30, and 48 in order to assess the association between the parents' level of education when the children were 8 years old and the children's subsequent well-being as they became adolescents and then adults. In a bivariate analysis comparing parents' education and subject's subsequent education, they found a significant association between the two. However, when they entered into the analysis the subjects' adolescent characteristics, the direct association between parents' education and children's subsequent education went away. As described by the authors, "the effects of parental education were entirely indirect: higher levels of parental education led to higher levels of optimistic educational aspirations or educational attainment in adolescence and subsequently to higher educational attainment or more prestigious occupational status in adulthood" (p. 240). It was the adolescent's own perspective on self-efficacy and the value of education that led her or him to continue with education after high school, with the resultant benefit in occupational status and the effects on well-being that status carries with it. The authors were able to determine that, as the single strongest predictor of subsequent educational attainment, what they refer to as "achievement-related aspirations" (p. 242) began to appear in middle school and continued into later adolescence. The authors also determined that these aspirations were affected by parents' level of education but not by family income independent of parental education.

Consistent with the data we examined in chapter 3 showing the consistent associations throughout adulthood between educational attainment and well-being, associations that are largely mediated by unhealthy behaviors such as smoking, diet, and exercise, Ross and Mirowsky (2011) analyzed data from a nationally representative sample of English-speaking adults in the United States between the ages of 19 and 95. They evaluated the association between the subject's level of education and the subject's current health status. Both the subject's own level of education and that of the subject's parents were associated with adult health status. The extent to which the subject smoked, was overweight, or failed to get regular exercise explained a large part of this association. They found, however, an additional factor that explained much of this association: the extent to which the subject developed a sense of control over his or her own life. Those who came out of childhood with a lower sense of control over the direction their life would take were both less likely to attain a higher level of education and more likely to engage in these unhealthy behaviors.

Nguyen et al. (2012) looked for this lack of a sense of control in a study of more than 15,000 adolescents in the United States. When the subjects were in the seventh through twelfth grades in school, researchers asked them to estimate their chances of living to age 35. They reinterviewed the subjects when they were 24–32 years old and evaluated their adult SES using measures of education, income, and life experiences. A lower estimate during adolescence of one's chances of surviving to age 35 was associated with a lower level of SES as an adult. Recalling the Present-Fatalistic and Present-Hedonistic time perspectives identified by Zimbardo and Boyd, as discussed in chapter 6, we can see consistent evidence that coming from a lower-SES family, in which parents had low levels of education and never passed on to their children a positive perspective on the potential of succeeding in school, can have profound impacts on the way an adolescent views the world and his or her place in it as well as the benefits or harms of adopting certain types of behavior in adolescence and as an adult. At such time as that adolescent becomes a parent, he or she is at risk of passing on to the next generation this fatalistic sense of low self-efficacy and the behavioral risks that go with it.

Summary

We have seen how adult well-being is closely tied to behaviors, including both those such as diet and smoking that are directly related to health status and to educational attainment as a fundamental correlate of these behaviors. The psychological and motivational factors that play a central role in determining these behaviors develop in childhood, especially early childhood.

Social inequality, whether economically or racially/ethnically based, can create high levels of stress for women giving birth to children and for their children. The impact of that stress on children's neural structure, cognitive functioning, and subsequent behavior is most acute during the pregnancy and in the first months and years of life. Based on the concept of "toxic stress," researchers have identified a range of adverse childhood outcomes that can be triggered by exposure during infancy to high levels of stress.

A principal outcome of that stress can be diminished readiness, both cognitively and behaviorally, when a child enters school. That lack of school readiness is commonly associated with lower educational performance during the early years of school and thus with the reduced perceptions of self-efficacy that often accompany weak performance. While some studies have documented that these adverse outcomes can be prevented through high-quality early childhood intervention, many of the children who enter kindergarten with impaired readiness will carry the consequences into adolescence and young adulthood. If the child is also a member of a disadvantaged racial or ethnic minority group, these consequences can be more profound. These issues raise the question of what types of interventions can be expected to prevent these outcomes in children who experience the toxic stress so often associated with economic or racial/ethnic inequality.

REFERENCES

Adverse Childhood Experiences Study, The. Described at http://acestudy.org/, accessed 8/8/14.

American Academy of Pediatrics. 2012. Policy statement: Early childhood adversity, toxic stress, and the role of the pediatrician: Translating developmental science into lifelong health. Pediatrics 129(1): e224-31.

———. 2014. Press release: American Academy of Pediatrics convenes thought leaders for symposium on reducing toxic stress and fostering resilience in children. June 12, available at www.aap.org/en-us/about-the-aap/aap-press-room/Pages/DCSymposium.aspx, accessed 7/31/14.

Bauldry, S., Shanahan, M. J., Boardman, J. D., Miech, R. A., & Macmillan, R. 2012. A life course model of self-rated health through adolescence and young adulthood. Social Science and Medicine 75(7): 1311-20.

Blair, R. J. R., Leibenluft, E., & Pine, D. S. 2014. Conduct disorder and callous-unemotional traits in youth. New England Journal of Medicine 371(23): 2207-16.

Bogart, L. M., Elliott, M. N., Kanouse, D. E., et al. 2013. Association between perceived discrimination and racial/ethnic disparities in problem behaviors among preadolescent youths. American Journal of Public Health 103(6): 1074-81.

Boyce, W. T., Obradovic, J., Bush, N. R., et al. 2012. Social stratification, classroom climate, and the behavioral adaptation of kindergarten children. Proceedings of the National Academy of Sciences USA 109(Supp. 2): 17168-73.

Boynton-Jarrett, R., Hair, E., & Zuckerman, B. 2013. Turbulent times: Effects of turbulence and violence exposure in adolescence on high school completion, health risk behavior, and mental health in young adulthood. Social Science and Medicine 95: 77-86.

Brooks, D. 2014. The character factory. New York Times, August 1, p. A21.

Center on the Developing Child at Harvard University. 2011. Building the brain's "air traffic control" system: How early experiences shape the development of executive function. Working Paper No. 11, available at www.developingchild.harvard.edu, accessed 8/4/14.

Davis-Kean, P. E. 2005. The influence of parent education and family income on child achievement: The indirect role of parental expectations and the home environment. Journal of Family Psychology 19(2): 294-304.

Dowd, J. B., Palermo, T., Chyu, L., Adam, E., & McDade, T. W. 2014. Race/ethnic and socioeconomic differences in stress and immune function in the National Longitudinal Study of Adolescent Health. Social Science and Medicine 115: 49-55.

Dubow, E. F., Boxer, P., & Huesmann, L. R. 2009. Long-term effects of parents' education on children's educational and occupational success mediation by family interactions, child aggression, and teenage aspirations. Merrill-Palmer Quarterly 55(3): 224-49.

Eccles, J. S., & Davis-Kean, P. E. 2005. Influences of parents' education on their children's educational attainments: The role of parent and child perceptions. London Review of Education 3(3): 191-204.

Francis, D. D. 2009. Conceptualizing child health disparities: A role for developmental neurogenomics. Pediatrics 124(Supp. 3): S196-202.

Fujimoto, K., & Valente, T. W. 2015. Multiplex congruity: Friendship networks and perceived popularity as correlates of adolescent alcohol use. Social Science and Medicine 125: 173-81.

Halfon, N. 2014. Socioeconomic influences on child health: Building new ladders of social opportunity. JAMA 311(9): 915-17.

Hanson, M. D., & Chen, E. 2007. Socioeconomic status and health behaviors in adolescence: A review of the literature. Journal of Behavioral Medicine 30(3): 263-85.

Heffernan, K. S., Jae, S. Y., Wilund, K. R., Woods, J. A., & Fernhall, B. 2008. Racial differences in central blood pressure and vascular function in young men. American Journal of Physiology Heart and Circulatory Physiology 295: H2380-87.

Institute of Medicine of the US National Academy of Sciences. 2001. Health and behavior: The interplay of biological, behavioral, and societal influences. Available at www.nap.edu/catalog.php?record_id =9838, accessed 7/28/14.

———. 2006. Genes, behavior, and the social environment: Moving beyond the nature/nurture debate. Available at www.nap.edu/catalog.php?record_id =11693, accessed 7/28/14.

Kamp Dush, C. M., Schmeer, K. K., & Taylor, M. 2013. Chaos as a social determinant of child health: Reciprocal associations? Social Science and Medicine 95: 69-76.

Luby, J., Belden, A., Botteron, K., et al. 2013. The effects of poverty on childhood brain development: The mediating effect of caregiving and stressful life events. JAMA Pediatrics 167(12): 1135-42.

Machado-de-Sousa, J. P., Osório, F. de L., Jackowski, A. P., et al. 2014. Increased amygdalar and hippocampal volumes in young adults with social anxiety. PLoS One 9(2): e88523.

McEwen, B. S. 1998. Protective and damaging effects of stress mediators. New England Journal of Medicine 338: 171-79.

———. 1999. Stress and hippocampal plasticity. Annual Review of Neurosciences 22: 105-22.

Murray, D. W., Rosanbalm, K., Christopoulos, C., & Hamoudi, A. 2015. Self-regulation and toxic stress: Foundations for understanding self-regulation from an applied developmental perspective. OPRE Report #2015-21. Washington, DC: Office of Planning, Research and Evaluation, Administration for Children and Families, US Department of Health and Human Services, available at www.acf.hhs.gov /sites/default/files/opre/report_1_foundations _paper_final_012715_submitted_0.pdf, accessed 3/7/15.

National Center for Education Statistics. 2001. Students whose parents did not go to college: Postsecondary access, persistence, and attainment, available at http://nces.ed.gov/pubs2001/2001126.pdf, accessed 8/7/14.

———. 2014. The condition of education: Status dropout rates, available at http://nces.ed.gov/programs/coe /indicator_coj.asp, accessed 8/7/14.

National Scientific Council on the Developing Child. 2014 [2005]. Excessive stress disrupts the architecture of the developing brain. Working Paper 3. Updated edition. Available at www.developingchild.harvard .edu, accessed 7/31/14.

Nelson, C. A. 2013. Biological embedding of early life adversity. JAMA Pediatrics 167(12): 1098-99.

Nguyen, Q. C., Hussey, J. M., Halpern, C. T., et al. 2012. Adolescent expectations of early death predict young adult socioeconomic status. Social Science and Medicine 74(9): 1452-60.

Noble, K. G., McCandliss, B. D., & Farah, M. J. 2007. Socioeconomic gradients predict individual differences in neurocognitive abilities. Developmental Science 10(4): 464-80.

Noble, K. G., Norman, M. F., & Farah, M. J. 2005. Neurocognitive correlates of socioeconomic status in kindergarten children. Developmental Science 8(1): 74-87.

Pachucki, M. C., Ozer, E. J., Barrat, A., & Cattuto, C. 2015. Mental health and social networks in early adolescence: A dynamic study of objectively-measured social interaction behaviors. Social Science and Medicine 125: 40-50.

Poonawalla, I. B., Kendzor, D. E., Owen, M. T., & Caughy, M. O. 2014. Family income trajectory during childhood is associated with adolescent cigarette smoking and alcohol use. Addictive Behaviors 39(10): 1383-8.

Portilla, X. A., Ballard, P. J., Adler, N. E., Boyce, W. T., & Obradović, J. 2014. An integrative view of school functioning: Transactions between self-regulation, school engagement, and teacher-child relationship quality. Child Development 85(5): 1915-31.

Priest, N., Paradies, Y., Trenerry, B., et al. 2013. A systematic review of studies examining the relationship between reported racism and health and wellbeing for children and young people. Social Science and Medicine 95: 115-27.

Qin, S., Young, C. B., Duan, X., et al. 2014. Amygdala subregional structure and intrinsic functional connectivity predicts individual differences in anxiety during early childhood. Biological Psychiatry 75(11): 892-900.

Rosen, J. 2014. Study: Children's life trajectories largely determined by family they are born into, available at http://hub.jhu.edu/2014/06/02/karl-alexander-long -shadow-research, accessed 8/7/14.

Ross, C. E., & Mirowsky, J. 2011. The interaction of personal and parental education on health. Social Science and Medicine 72(4): 591-99.

Sanders-Phillips, K., Settles-Reaves, B., Walker, D., & Brownlow, J. 2009. Social inequality and racial discrimination: Risk factors for health disparities in children of color. Pediatrics 124(Supp. 3): S176-86.

Seeman, T., Epel, E., Gruenewald, T., Karlamangla, A., & McEwen, B. S. 2010. Socio-economic differentials in peripheral biology: Cumulative allostatic load. Annals of the New York Academy of Sciences 1186: 223-39.

Shonkoff, J. P. 2003. From neurons to neighborhoods: Old and new challenges for developmental and behavioral pediatrics. Journal of Developmental and Behavioral Pediatrics 24(1): 70-76.

———. 2012. Leveraging the biology of adversity to address the roots of disparities in health and development. Proceedings of the National Academy of Sciences USA 109(Supp. 2): 17302-7.

Shonkoff, J. P., Boyce, W. T., & McEwen, B. S. 2009. Neuroscience, molecular biology, and the childhood roots of health disparities: Building a new framework for health promotion and disease prevention. JAMA 301(21): 2252-59.

Shonkoff, J. P., Garner, A. S., et al. 2012. The lifelong effects of early childhood adversity and toxic stress. Pediatrics 129(1): e232-46.

Shonkoff, J. P., & Phillips, D. A., Eds. 2000. From Neurons to Neighborhoods: The Science of Early Childhood Development. National Academy Press, available at www.nap.edu/catalog.php?record_id=9824, accessed 5/12/14.

Thurston, R. C., & Matthews, K. A. 2009. Racial and socioeconomic disparities in arterial stiffness and intima media thickness among adolescents. Social Science and Medicine 68: 807-13.

Welsh, J. A., Nix, R. L., Blair, C., Bierman, K. L., & Nelson, K. E. 2010. The development of cognitive skills and gains in academic school readiness for children from low-income families. Journal of Educational Psychology 102(1): 43-53.

World Health Organization. 2009. Addressing adverse childhood experiences to improve public health. Meeting Report, available at www.who.int/violence _injury_prevention/violence/activities/adverse _childhood_experiences/global_research_network _may_2009.pdf, accessed 8/8/14.

CHAPTER 11

Understanding Well-Being
and the Interventions
That Can Enhance It

In 2010, officials from the World Health Organization and the
US Centers for Disease Control and Prevention, working with
researchers with the Adverse Child Experiences (ACE) Study,
announced a collaborative effort to initiate a global surveillance
program to gauge the incidence and lifelong effects of ACEs (Anda
et al. 2010). They recommended that the public health community
adopt a new perspective on ACEs, approaching them as a potentially preventable problem. As they described, "The concept in
using ACEs as a framework for the primary prevention of public
health problems is that stressful or traumatic childhood experiences
such as abuse, neglect, or forms of household dysfunction are a
common pathway to social, emotional, and cognitive impairments
that lead to increased risk of unhealthy behaviors, violence or revic-
timization, disease, disability, and premature mortality" (p. 95).

Figure 11.1, adapted from the ACE Study website, describes
graphically the potentially lifelong effects of ACE on social, emotional, and cognitive functioning. These functional changes are
often associated with alterations in neurological structure, in particular in the hippocampus, amygdala, and associated cortical areas.
During childhood and adolescence these changes increase the likelihood that individuals experiencing ACEs will adopt behaviors that
put their current and future health at risk. These behaviors include
smoking, diet, and sexual activity but in particular also include
a child's response to educational challenges and opportunities.

Anda et al. emphasize the long-term impacts of events occurring early in childhood: "Although such events constitute a key
target for preventive attention, only a small fraction have acute
consequences of sufficient severity to bring them to the attention
of public authorities. By far, the largest proportion of the burden
of disease due to ACEs arises from the cumulative effect of

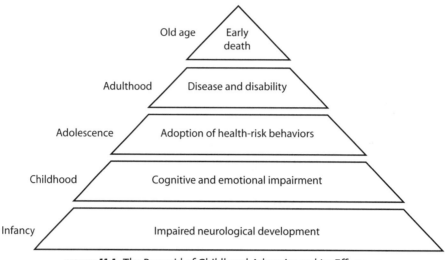

FIGURE 11.1. The Pyramid of Childhood Adversity and Its Effects on Well-Being. From the Adverse Childhood Experiences Study.

chronic exposure to multiple adversities whose lifelong consequences may often start to become apparent only many years after exposure" (p. 95). For example, while smoking is a principal cause both of premature death among many population groups and of persisting socioeconomic differences in life expectancy and quality of life, the root causes of adult smoking may actually occur in early childhood. The same is often true for the patterns of diet and exercise one adopts as an adult.

The previous chapters have described many of the processes involved in these developmental changes, from early development of the brain with selective axonal myelination to the development of cognitive abilities such as language and memory and the development of certain personality characteristics and associated motivational patterns. Again as described by Anda et al., "Breakthroughs in neurobiology show that ACEs disrupt neurodevelopment and have lasting effects on brain structure and function" (p. 95). As the pyramid in figure 11.1 suggests, these early developmental processes can have continuing impacts on well-being, both emotional and physical, at all stages of life from childhood through old age.

Social inequalities in adult health

In chapters 2 and 3 we discussed the many ways to measure health inequality and the ways health inequality is linked to socioeconomic inequality. We know, for example, that among adults in the United States age 60 or greater, lower income and lower levels of education are associated both with greater frequency of many chronic illnesses and with greater limitations in the level of physical functioning compared to others with comparable disease burdens (Louie and Ward 2011).

Similar outcomes exist for racial and ethnic minority groups. Exploring the association of chronically stressful adult living conditions and health outcomes, Jackson et al. concluded that, "Many Black Americans live in chronically precarious and difficult environments. These environments produce stressful living conditions, and often the most easily accessible options for addressing stress are various unhealthy behaviors . . . [that] have direct and debilitating effects on physical health" (2009, p. 936). Shariff-Marco et al. (2010) confirmed that among black Americans, having experienced racial discrimination is an added stressor that increases the risk for unhealthy behaviors.

It is becoming increasingly clear that behaviors adopted at an early age will continue to have powerful health impacts throughout the life course, including in old age. Shaw et al. (2013) tracked rates of death and disability over a 10-year period in a nationally representative sample of nearly 20,000 adults over the age of 50, all of whom were free of disability at the beginning of the study. As we would expect, they found significant disparities in these outcomes in association with socioeconomic status, although these disparities became somewhat smaller in the older age groups. Those disparities were significantly reduced, however, after they took into account behavioral patterns that were present at the beginning of the study. As the authors concluded, "This finding indicates that while the aging process is associated with some degree of leveling of socioeconomic inequalities, it is not enough to overcome the inequalities in health behaviors and health outcomes that have already accumulated" (Shaw et al. 2013, p. 57).

The early roots of adult health behaviors

If health behaviors in the middle years of life continue to impact health status into old age, how early are the roots of these behaviors established? The pyramid shown in figure 11.1 suggests that the origins of health-related behaviors are in adolescence. These adolescent behaviors, however, may have roots in early childhood, especially if that childhood included ACEs. Is there evidence that the health status of adults is linked directly to early childhood circumstances?

One of the earliest studies that provides data to address this question was begun in 1921 by Lewis Terman, one of the creators of the Stanford-Binet IQ test. As described in chapter 7, Terman identified 1,285 children with an average age of about 11 years, all of whom had an IQ of 135 or greater based on that test. These children were nearly all white and from middle-class families. Schwartz et al. (1995) reported follow-up data on this sample through the year 1991. By that time, 44 percent of the subjects had died. The authors looked at four aspects of the subjects' childhood experiences: family socioeconomic status (SES), health status during childhood, personality characteristics during childhood, and family stability. They assessed how these characteristics were associated with the risk of dying before 1991.

As we would expect, the girls in the study had a lower mortality rate over the 70 years of follow-up. Given the relative homogeneity of the subjects' socioeconomic status, researchers did not find a significant association between family SES and mortality risk. They did find that those subjects who as children exhibited the personality traits of conscientiousness and mood stability had lower rates of death. Beyond these associations, the only factor associated with an increased risk of death was having experienced parental divorce before the age of 21. Those children whose parents had divorced experienced a 44 percent increase in their mortality risk over the period of the study. Based on these findings, the authors pose an important question: "What are the precise causal mechanisms responsible for the associations between childhood personality, parental divorce, and longevity? This question is difficult to answer. The causal pathways probably involve the interaction of a number of factors, including health-related behaviors, stress and coping mechanisms, social support, and other lifestyle factors" (Schwartz et al. 1995, p. 1244)

Friedman et al. (1995) looked further at the association identified in the Terman study between the level of conscientiousness exhibited as a child and the cause of death for those subjects who had died between 1950 and 1986. The child's level of conscientiousness was based on reports obtained in 1922 from the child's parent and the child's teacher regarding four aspects of personality: prudence, conscientiousness, freedom from vanity/egotism, and truthfulness. The authors of this report suggest that this measure corresponds fairly closely to the Big Five dimension of conscientiousness, as discussed in chapter 7. They found that those children who exhibited higher levels of this trait as children were, as adults, less likely to smoke or drink heavily, although childhood conscientiousness remained strongly associated with longevity even after controlling for these behaviors.

Crosnoe and Elder (2004) looked at a subset of the men from the Terman study who were still alive in the 1970s. At the time of the update the subjects would have been between 63 and 72 years of age. The researchers created a scale of what they referred to as a holistic pattern of aging, which was essentially a global measure of subjects' overall quality of life. Factors included in this measure were current family engagement, perceived occupational success, civic involvement, life satisfaction, and vitality. They found that three aspects of childhood were associated with a holistic aging pattern in later years: the socioeconomic status of the family in which the child grew up, whether the subject's parents divorced during the subject's childhood, and the strength of the subject's attachment to her or his parents during childhood. From these results the authors were able to conclude that "early experiences can have long-term consequences . . . elements of earlier life stages, including family experiences, provide information about the routes that individuals take through life" (p. 650). An additional finding from this analysis was that the association between the socioeconomic situation of a subject's childhood family and the quality of the subject's aging profile in later life "was almost completely a function of the greater educational attainment of young people who grew up in such families" (p. 649).

A second group of studies that linked early childhood personality traits with adult health behaviors and health outcomes was done by Hampson, Goldberg, and colleagues (Hampson et al. 2006, 2007). As described in chapter 7, these data, originally gathered between 1959 and 1967, assessed the personality characteristics of elementary school children in Hawaii based on the Big Five traits model. When behaviors and health status were then reassessed when the subjects were in their 40s, researchers found that greater conscientiousness as a child was once again associated with greater adult quality of life, reduced rates of smoking, and reduced rates of obesity. These associations were stronger for women than for men. As with the Terman study, educational attainment played an important mediating role in the association between childhood conscientiousness and adult health behaviors.

Moffitt et al. (2011) reported on a longitudinal study of approximately 1,000 children born in 1972-73 in a city in New Zealand, who were followed to the age of 32. At age 5 years, children were observed by a trained examiner who rated them on a combined scale of self-control. Researchers then evaluated the association between self-control at age 5 and a range of indicators of well-being at age 32, including measures of physical health, mental health, wealth, and having a record of criminal activity. After controlling for childhood measurements of intelligence, socioeconomic status, and quality of family life, they found that self-control as a child was strongly associated with each of these measures of adult well-being.

Ferguson et al. (2005a, 2005b) reported on another longitudinal study of children in New Zealand. The study followed 1,265 children, all born in 1977, from birth through age 25. Using reports from parents and teachers, between the ages of 7 and 9 they measured the child's intelligence using a standardized IQ test as well as the child's "tendencies to disruptive, oppositional, and conduct disordered behaviours." They then evaluated the association between these measures taken at age 7 with two sets of outcomes assessed between age 18 and age 25: (1) education and employment and (2) adverse social out-

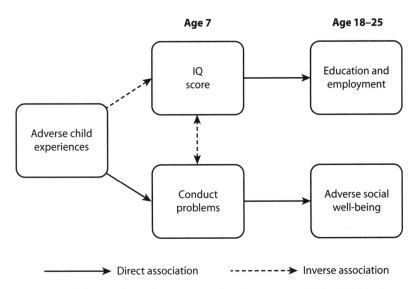

Age 7   **Age 18–25**

FIGURE 11.2. Association between Conduct Problems and IQ in Childhood with Educational and Social Outcomes in Early Adulthood in a Longitudinal Study of Children in New Zealand. From Ferguson et al. 2005a, 2005b.

comes, which included a history of criminal activity, drug abuse, mental illness, or unstable sexual or partner relationships. In their analyses they also included a measure of early ACEs, which included family conflict, socioeconomic adversity, parental instability, and violence or child abuse. The results of these studies are shown in figure 11.2.

As can be seen, early experience of ACEs was associated with lower IQ at age 7 and a greater frequency of conduct problems as assessed by both parents and teachers. These two outcomes were inversely associated, with children with higher IQs exhibiting fewer conduct problems. The child's IQ score at age 7 was a significant predictor of subsequent educational attainment and employment, while the level of conduct problems was significantly associated with greater social adversity as a young adult. In their full analysis, after accounting for conduct problems, there was no direct association between IQ and subsequent social adversity.

Bethell et al. (2014) studied data from the National Survey of Children's Health, which sur-

veyed a nationally representative sample of nearly 100,000 children between the ages of 0 and 17. Using data gathered in 2011-12 and controlling for demographic characteristics, they found that those children and adolescents reporting a greater frequency of ACEs had both lower school engagement and higher rates of chronic illnesses such as asthma, obesity, and ADHD. They also found that those children who, between the ages of 6 and 17, displayed what the authors refer to as "resilience" (defined as "staying calm and in control when faced with a challenge") showed fewer adverse impacts of earlier ACEs.

In chapter 9 we discussed the development of memory and other forms of cognition, describing them largely in terms of the neural structure of certain regions of the brain. If (a) the children in the Terman study with lower levels of conscientiousness subsequently also showed lower levels of educational attainment, (b) the children in the Moffit study who showed less self-control had reduced well-being in their thirties, and (c) the children in the Ferguson study with more conduct problems exhibited lower levels of intelligence and subsequent educational attainment, might the children in these studies have had lower levels of cognitive functioning as a contributor to these differences? Evans and Schamberg (2009) addressed this issue in a study of 195 young adults who were part of a longitudinal study of rural poverty. The subjects were white and 50 percent female, with half in families living below the poverty line and half living in middle class families with incomes 2–4 times the poverty line. The subjects were followed from birth through age 17, with regular assessment of the family's poverty status and measures of allostatic load, the body's physiologic stress response (e.g., blood pressure, level of stress hormones). When the subjects were an average age of 17.3 years, they had their working memory assessed using a standard psychological assessment. When the researchers only assessed the association between the length of time living in poverty and working memory at age 17, they found a significant inverse association. When they included both the time in poverty and the allostatic load in the analysis, the allostatic load was inversely associated with working memory, while poverty no longer showing an association with memory. By the time they are 17 years old, young adults who, as children, experienced the stress of poverty have developed less cognitive capacity for working memory. Those with less cognitive capacity at this age are less likely to continue education beyond high school and are accordingly likely to experience reduced earning capacity and more likely to engage as adults in behaviors that reduce their well-being. In a study of poor adults in an urban setting in the United States and in a rural setting in India, Mani et al. (2013) confirmed this association between continued poverty and reduced cognitive functioning as adults.

In a commentary responding to the Moffit study of self-control during childhood, Duckworth suggested that "Self-controlled individuals are more adept than their counterparts at regulating their behavioral, emotional, and attentional impulses to achieve long-term goals . . . The benefits of self-control for adult functioning are partially mediated by better decision making during adolescence" (2011, p. 2639).

Adler and Snibbe (2003) have reviewed research in sociology and psychology about the factors that create the long-term association between socioeconomic status and health. They show how this association begins in childhood, with the social and economic context in which the child grows up affecting the development of personality traits and cognitive abilities. These in turn are associated with both physiologic consequences of allostatic load and the health-relevant behaviors adopted in adolescence. They suggest that a key linkage between reduced socioeconomic circumstances and subsequent adverse health outcomes is to a large extent a consequence of "Behavioral, cognitive, and affective tendencies that develop in response to the greater psychosocial stress encountered in low-SES environments" (p. 119). They also conclude that "Extensive data attest to the centrality of perceived personal control and mastery in the SES-health gradient" (p. 120). In their report, Adler and Snibbe provide a graphic representation of the longitudinal succession of factors, from childhood through adolescence, that affect health and well-being as adults. Their model includes environmental factors in addition to psychological factors. In figure 11.3 I have reproduced that portion of their diagram that focuses on psychological factors.

In comparing figure 11.3, adapted from Adler and Snibbe, to figure 11.1, from the Adverse Childhood Experiences Study, we see essentially the same causal chain, only using a different axis to represent time. Data from a range of studies, done over a range of time periods following a range of populations, have confirmed the causal linkages represented in both diagrams.

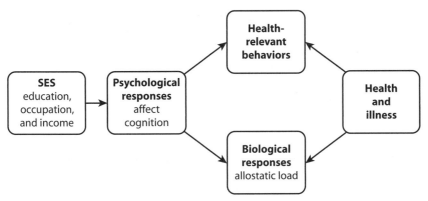

FIGURE 11.3. The Pathways from Socioeconomic Status to Health. Adapted from Adler and Snibbe 2003.

A review of the impacts of social determinants concluded, "Research shows that early life exposures affect cognitive and noncognitive development (for example, executive function and prefrontal cortex development), which, in turn, affects time preferences and self-control skills (delayed gratification), which are major determinants of risky health behaviors. These are key neuro-psycho-social pathways connecting socioeconomic status, health behavior, and health outcomes" (Health Policy Brief 2014).

Identifying and adopting interventions to improve adult health through the reduction of adverse childhood experiences

In one of the early publications from the ACE Study, Felitti et al. summarized the implications of the causal linkages illustrated above: "These associations are important because it is now clear that the leading causes of morbidity and mortality in the United States are related to health behaviors and lifestyle factors; these factors have been called the 'actual' causes of death. Insofar as abuse and other potentially damaging childhood experiences contribute to the development of these risk factors, then these childhood exposures should be recognized as

the basic causes of morbidity and mortality in adult life" (1998, p. 246).

If the cognitive deficit that is the consequence of early childhood adversity leads to reduced educational attainment and to behaviors that are harmful to health, then it makes sense to view childhood adversity as a cause of premature death in later adulthood. As described at the beginning of this chapter, the World Health Organization and the US Centers for Disease Control and Prevention have jointly called for a new international perspective on the implications of ACEs (Anda et al. 2010). In much the same way as public health agencies have collaborated globally to follow and reduce infectious diseases, these agencies called for "a framework for global surveillance of the prevalence and broad public impact of ACEs" (p. 96).

As with any global health issue that has a long chain of causal and contributory factors, it is not always clear at what point in that chain it would be optimal to intervene. It would be shortsighted to suggest that attempting to change adverse health behaviors of adults who have already begun to develop signs of chronic illness would be most effective. Rigotti et al. (2014) reported on a trial studying 397 adults who had been hospitalized for treatment of an acute problem, most commonly related to cardiovascular disease, all of whom had been daily smokers before their hospitalization. The patients, with an average age of 53 years, were randomly assigned either to receive a sustained smoking cessation intervention upon discharge from the hospital or to receive standard advice about the importance of quitting smoking and the availability of medications to assist with quitting. The sustained intervention included a free 90-day supply of tobacco cessation medication, regular automated phone calls to encourage them to refrain from smoking, and the availability of a counselor to contact for further assistance in stopping smoking. While there was a slight increase in the percentage of participants who received the sustained intervention who had stopped smoking at six months after discharge (25% for the intervention group as compared to 15% for the standard care group), three-fourths of these patients with a known, potentially serious chronic medical condition for which smoking was a major contributory factor nonetheless continued to smoke despite the intensive intervention. Similar results have been found in intensive efforts to reduce obesity among adults with diabetes and other conditions related to obesity (Wadden et al. 2014).

Another possible place to intervene might be at the point where individuals end their education. Kulhánová et al. (2014) used mortality data from countries in Western Europe to do a mathematical estimate of the effect on adult mortality if everyone in those countries were to complete some form of higher education after high school. Perhaps not surprisingly, mortality would be reduced as much as 50 percent for both men and women in some countries. In the United States, as in these Western European countries, experience has shown that this hypothetical output cannot be easily attained. While government agencies, school districts, and educational researchers have tried a number of interventions to increase rates of high school completion followed by participation in higher education, levels of educational attainment remain low for many groups.

The effects of early childhood intervention for children at risk of ACEs

As we saw in chapter 3, African Americans have some of the highest death rates, lowest life expectancy, lowest educational attainment levels, and highest rates of risky health behaviors of all racial/ethnic groups in the United States. Many of these disparities are due to the lower socioeconomic circumstances in which many black children grow up, compounded by the stress of experiencing racial discrimination. Adopting the causal model of the ACE Study, would it be possible to prevent the chain of adverse cognitive, behavioral, and health outcomes experienced by many African Americans throughout the developmental process?

Reynolds et al. (2014) studied nearly 1,000 mostly low-income, single-parent preschool children in Chicago, 90 percent of whom were black and 7 percent of whom were Hispanic. Forty-two percent of the children attended preschool full-time (seven hours per day), while 58 percent attended preschool for three hours per day. The researchers used a case-control methodology to determine if full-day preschool had greater benefits for the children than part-day. They found that attending full-day preschool was associated with higher scores on scales of school readiness that measured language ability, math ability, socioemotional development, and physical health. In addition, the full-day students showed increased attendance rates and reduced chronic absences. In an editorial that accompanied the study by Reynolds, Schweinhart commented that studies on the value of preschool "generally have supported the idea that greater program quality and quantity, such as full-day vs. part-day, contribute more to children's development" (2014, p. 2101)

A group of researchers at the University of North Carolina, Chapel Hill, also explored the value of full-day preschool. In what they have described as the Carolina Abecedarian Project, they asked this question in regard to the value of preschool for children starting shortly after birth. Beginning in 1972, researchers enrolled the families of 104 newborn infants, evenly split between boys and girls and all from families living in the Chapel Hill area of North Carolina. The families were identified as high risk based on a series of criteria that included meeting poverty guidelines defined by the federal government; the age and educational level of the mother (average age 20 years, average educational attainment 10th grade); and family structure (75% single-parent households). Based on these criteria and the region from which families were recruited, 98 percent of the infants were African American, although race was not used as an explicit selection criterion.

The children were randomized at birth, with half of the children receiving intensive social and educational support beginning at birth. The intervention included full-time, year-round professional day care for five days per week from birth to age 5. The program in the day care included age-appropriate interventions to teach basic cognitive and social skills as well as frequent interaction that emphasized the development of language skills. Those children randomized to the control group received no specialized intervention, although some children did participate in existing day care programs in the area. Families from both groups were offered social service support that they could call on if needed.

The intervention ended when the children reached age 5 and were ready to enter school. At that point, a second randomization took place, with each of the two original groups (intervention and control) further split into one group that would receive an additional intervention during the first three years of school and another that would experience the standard school curriculum. The families in the school intervention group, half of which had participated in the early childhood intervention and half of which had not, were assigned a trained home-resource teacher to supplement the usual grade-level school teacher. For the first three years of

school, this resource teacher acted as a liaison between the family and the school and developed individual, supplementary curriculum packets for the children based on their learning needs as identified by the classroom teacher.

The researchers then evaluated children on a regular basis, beginning at age 3, comparing the cognitive and academic development of the children (Campbell et al. 2001). When the subjects were 21 years old, they were compared based on their intellectual and academic abilities, their level of educational attainment, their level of employment, and their overall social adjustment (Campbell et al. 2002). When the subjects in the study had reached their mid-30s, they were then compared on a range of risk factors for cardiovascular and other metabolic diseases (Campbell et al. 2014). The comparative outcomes between the early childhood intervention group and the control group at these various ages are shown in table 11.1. The table only shows the outcomes that were shown to be associated with the early childhood intervention portion of the study. In most cases, the three-year school-age intervention did not have additional impacts beyond those of the early intervention.

These studies identified a number of significant impacts of the early childhood intervention. These impacts were apparent by the age of 3 and continued to be apparent when the subjects were in their mid-30s.

As shown in table 11.1, the differences in outcomes of the children receiving the intervention as compared to those who did not included the following:

- At age 3 to age 5, the study subjects had greater cognitive ability as measured by a standard IQ test.
- At age 8 and age 15, the study subjects continued to have greater cognitive ability, and they had developed greater reading and math ability.
- At age 21, the study subjects continued to display greater cognitive and academic

ability, had better educational attainment, and showed evidence of better social adjustment based on a range of behaviors.

- By their mid-30s, the study subjects had evidence of better physical health based on a range of physiologic risk markers.

A second long-term study of the impact of high quality preschool on the lives of children

born into disadvantaged circumstances largely corroborated the conclusions of the Abecedarian study. The High/Scope Perry Preschool study was begun in 1962 and involved 123 children from low-income black families living in Ypsilanti, Michigan (Schweinhart et al. 2005). The children were randomly assigned either to receive a high-quality preschool program at age 3 through 4 or no preschool program. The pre-

TABLE 11.1. Comparative Outcomes of the Early Childhood Intervention in the Abecedarian Project

Outcome measured	Evaluation results			
	3–5 years			
	Study		**Control**	
Cognitive ability (IQ score)	101.3		89.2	
	8 years		**15 years**	
	Study	**Control**	**Study**	**Control**
Cognitive ability (IQ score)	97.8	93.8	95.8	90.1
Reading ability (test score)	94.0	85.2	94.3	88.5
Math ability (test score)	97.7	92.5	93.6	86.8
	21 years			
Cognitive/academic	**Study**		**Control**	
Cognitive ability (IQ score)	89.7		85.2	
Reading ability (test score)	93.3		87.6	
Math ability (test score)	89.2		84.5	
Educational attainment				
Graduated high school	70%		67%	
Enrolled in college	36%		14%	
Social adjustment				
Currently employed	64%		50%	
Married	4%		10%	
Teenage parent	26%		45%	
Regular smoker	39%		55%	
	Mid-30s			
Adult health indicator	**Study**		**Control**	
High blood pressure	22%		32%	
Elevated cholesterol	28%		46%	
Diabetes or prediabetes	35%		36%	
Obesity	67%		77%	

Sources: Campbell et al. 2001, 2002, 2014.
Note: Study group received intervention from birth to 5 years; control group received no early intervention.

school experience was offered by fully certified teachers, each working with groups of five to six children. There was a daily class schedule, and the teacher visited each child's family once a week.

The researchers followed 94 percent of the children into their 40s, assessing their educational progress and socioeconomic status on a regular basis. From these analyses they have identified a number of significant differences in the life courses of the two groups of children.

- At age 5, the preschool children had higher average IQ.
- At age 14–15, the preschool children showed more consistent completion of homework and had demonstrated better academic achievement.
- More of the preschool children than nonpreschool children graduated from high school (77% vs. 60%).
- At age 40, the preschool children showed higher incomes and had been arrested fewer times.

The results of both the Abecedarian study and the Perry Preschool study confirm the causal linkages shown both in the model from the ACE study included in figure 11.1 and in the model proposed by Adler and Snibbe shown in figure 11.3. Many chronic disease risks and the behaviors that contribute to them are, to a substantial degree, the consequence of the circumstances in which a child was raised. Those raised in supportive, socioeconomically advantaged circumstances are more likely to develop early cognitive abilities that are conducive to educational success. These abilities, in combination with the personality and motivational characteristics of the child as he or she moves through adolescence into adulthood, will be associated with behavioral patterns that are conducive to continued educational success and to the reduced risk for chronic illness associated with that success. By contrast, those children who experience adverse circumstances early in childhood are likely to develop weaker cognitive abilities and to develop personality and motivational characteristics that put them at risk for risky behaviors and less educational success. These outcomes place these children at increased risk as adults of developing chronic illness and succumbing to early mortality. The most effective time to intervene in this causal chain is at its beginning, in the period immediately following birth. James Heckman (2006) performed a cost/benefit analysis of investing public resources in early childhood education and support programs and concluded that "The benefit-cost ratio (the ratio of the aggregate program benefits over the life of the child to the input costs) is over eight to one" (p. 1901). By contrast, Heckman estimates, investing in changing educational and health-related behaviors in high school and adulthood yields substantially less than the cost of the public resources required.

Home visitors and the Maternal, Infant, and Early Childhood Home Visiting Program

Based on growing awareness of the significance of early childhood experiences on subsequent development, with direct consequences for educational attainment, health risk behaviors, and well-being during adulthood, the medical and public health communities have been paying increasing attention to developing programs to identify children at risk for ACEs based on family structure and dynamics. Consistent with the findings of the Abecedarian study, substantial emphasis has been given to developing early intervention programs, many beginning at or even before birth, to mitigate the effects of an adverse home environment. Many of these efforts involve a home visitor, often a nurse or other trained professional, who meets the parents in the home context to provide education, support, and counseling to the family. Some of these are also linked to preschool programs.

Howard and Brookes-Gunn (2009) reviewed the outcomes from a range of home-visitor programs, mostly targeting children born into families at risk for abuse or other adverse parenting behaviors. From this review, the authors were able to conclude that "evidence is mounting that these programs can positively alter parenting practices and, to a lesser extent, children's cognitive development" (p. 138). The mixed outcomes in affecting children's cognitive development may have been due to the heterogeneity of the program designs and the fact that relatively few of these programs included high-quality day care that emphasized language and cognitive development.

Brennan et al. (2013) looked specifically at the potential benefit of working with the parents of young children born into circumstances that placed them at high risk of developing future behavior problems. The authors based their study on previous research demonstrating that "parenting practices during the early childhood period, when child regulatory strategies and problem-solving approaches are being established, [are] critical in setting up the cognitive and behavioral foundations with which children enter school" (p. 763).

The authors identified 731 children in low-income, potentially high-risk families in three metropolitan areas: Pittsburgh, Pennsylvania, Eugene, Oregon, and Charlottesville, Virginia. When the children were 2 years old, approximately half of the families were randomly assigned to receive a series of "family check-ups," in which a trained parenting consultant met with the primary caregiver of each child three times over a period of a few weeks to discuss optimal approaches to parenting a young child, encouraging the caregiver to adopt what the researchers referred to as a "positive behavior support" model of parenting. The caregivers in the intervention group received a yearly family check-up when their child was 2, 3, 4, and 5 years old. When they were assessed at ages 5 and 7.5, the children in the intervention group had significantly better aca-

demic achievement than the control group who did not receive the check-ups, leading the authors to conclude that "a brief, parenting-focused intervention during early childhood may be a viable strategy to prevent at-risk children from developing behavior problems and low academic achievement at school age" (p. 769).

In 2009, the American Academy of Pediatrics published a report developed by its Council on Community Pediatrics about the role of early childhood programs that involve home visitors. Based on the council's review of the available evidence, it concluded that "Home-visiting programs offer a mechanism for ensuring that at-risk families have social support, linkage with public and private community services, and ongoing health, developmental, and safety education. When these services are part of a system of high-quality well-child care linked or integrated with the pediatric medical home, they have the potential to mitigate health and developmental outcome disparities" (p. 598).

Largely in response to the growing body of evidence in support of the potential value of home visitor programs, the Affordable Care Act (ACA), signed into law by President Obama in 2010, included funding for a new national program to expand the availability of and to evaluate the effectiveness of home visitor programs for mothers of young children in at-risk families. ACA amended Title V of the Social Security Act to create the Maternal, Infant, and Early Childhood Home Visiting Program, allocating $1.5 billion for fiscal years 2010–14 to be used by states, territories, and tribes to expand home visiting programs.

ACA also created the Mother and Infant Home Visiting Program Evaluation (MIHOPE), mandating that the federal Department of Health and Human Services initiate an ongoing assessment of the effectiveness of these programs in several states and report the findings to Congress on a regular basis. The first report was issued in January of 2015 (Michalopoulos et al. 2015). As described in this report,

MIHOPE has included four different models of current home visiting programs in its analysis: Early Head Start—Home Based Program Option, Healthy Families America, Nurse-Family Partnership, and Parents as Teachers. It selected 88 of these programs drawn from 12 states to include in its evaluation.

The initial report in 2015 provides data on the demographics of the families served by these programs. Assessment of actual program outcomes will come in later reports. The average age of the women enrolled in the programs was 23; 70 percent of these women were pregnant. More than half of these pregnant women were under age 21. As would be expected based on the risk selection, the participants in the study were disproportionately from a lower socioeconomic position, with 92 percent receiving public assistance such as cash welfare payments. More than 75 percent of the women in the study had not finished high school, and about 1 in 10 reported having been the victim of intimate partner violence. Consistent with these risk factors, more than 30 percent of the women reported symptoms of depression. As might be also be expected based on these socioeconomic characteristics, the sample is disproportionately nonwhite: 34 percent are Hispanic, 31 percent black, and 25 percent white.

The report describes the principal outcomes it will be assessing over time in these programs: parent and child health, child development, parenting skills, school readiness and academic achievement, crime or domestic violence, and family economic self-sufficiency. As future reports compare these outcomes among the different program models, we will have a stronger sense of which types of home visitor programs hold the most promise for future investment.

Looking to the future

In December 2011, the Arthur M. Sackler Colloquium of the National Academy of Sciences sponsored an international scientific meeting titled "Biological Embedding of Early Social Adversity: From Fruit Flies to Kindergartners." At that meeting, Michael Rutter of the Medical Research Council of Kings College London summarized the issues facing developmental scientists:

> The starting point for the study of adverse experiences is that some have enduring consequences that continue after the period of exposure to the adversity. That raises four basic issues: whether social adversities can be considered homogeneous, whether the crucial effect lies in the 'objective' or subjectively perceived 'effective' environment, whether the effects are environmentally mediated, and whether the form of biological embedding involves psychological or health consequences. (Rutter 2012, p. 17149)

While there is a great deal of information available about various aspects of the child development process, how development is affected by the environment in which a child is raised, how the outcomes of that process affect educational attainment and other aspects of behavior, and how these in turn affect lifetime well-being, the questions Rutter poses have not yet been fully addressed. Given the growing attention to the issue of human behavior and how it affects well-being, we can expect to see important new data regarding these issues becoming available in the next several years. The research will be in the areas of biology, psychology, sociology, and other related disciplines. As I have suggested throughout this book, the most fruitful advances in our understanding of these issues may come as a result of approaching the issue of human behavior from a perspective that integrates these traditionally distinct disciplines and by focusing on the early childhood experience as perhaps the most appropriate time for intervention.

REFERENCES

Adler, N. E., & Snibbe, A. C. 2003. The role of psychosocial processes in explaining the gradient between socioeconomic status and health. Current Directions in Psychological Science 12(4): 119-23.

American Academy of Pediatrics, Council on Community Pediatrics. 2009. The role of preschool home-visiting programs in improving children's developmental and health outcomes. Pediatrics 123(2): 598-603.

Anda, R. F., Butchart, A., Felitti, V. J., & Brown, D. W. 2010. Building a framework for global surveillance of the public health implications of adverse childhood experiences. American Journal of Preventive Medicine 39(1): 93-98.

Bethell, C. D., Newacheck, P., Hawes, E., & Halfon, N. 2014. Adverse childhood experiences: Assessing the impact on health and school engagement and the mitigating role of resilience. Health Affairs 33(12): 2106-15.

Brennan, L. M., Shelleby, E. C., Shaw, D. S., et al. 2013. Indirect effects of the family check-up on school-age academic achievement through improvements in parenting in early childhood. Journal of Educational Psychology 105(3): 762-73.

Campbell, F., Conti, G., Heckman, J. J., et al. 2014. Early childhood investments substantially boost adult health. Science 343(6178): 1478-85.

Campbell, F. A., Pungello, E. P., Miller-Johnson, S., Burchinal, M., & Ramey, C. T. 2001. The development of cognitive and academic abilities: Growth curves from an early childhood educational experiment. Developmental Psychology 37(2): 231-42.

Campbell, F. A., Ramey, C. T., Pungello, E., Sparling, J., & Miller-Johnson, S. 2002. Early childhood education: Young adult outcomes from the Abecedarian project. Applied Developmental Science 6(1): 42-57.

Carolina Abecedarian Project, The. Described at http://abc.fpg.unc.edu/, accessed 8/21/14.

Crosnoe, R., & Elder, G. H. Jr. 2004. From childhood to later years: Pathways of human development. Research on Aging 26(6): 623-54.

Duckworth A. L. 2011. The significance of self-control. Proceedings of the National Academy of Sciences USA 108(7): 2639-40.

Evans, G. W., & Schamberg, M. A. 2009. Childhood poverty, chronic stress, and adult working memory. Proceedings of the National Academy of Sciences USA 106(16): 6545-49.

Felitti, V. J., Anda, R. F., Nordenberg, D., et al. 1998. Relationship of childhood abuse and household dysfunction to many of the leading causes of death in adults: The Adverse Childhood Experiences (ACE) Study. American Journal of Preventive Medicine 14(4): 245-58.

Ferguson, D. M., Horwood, L. J., & Ridder, E. M. 2005a. Show me the child at seven: The consequences of conduct problems in childhood for psychosocial functioning in adulthood. Journal of Child Psychology and Psychiatry 46(8): 837-49.

———. 2005b. Show me the child at seven II: Childhood intelligence and later outcomes in adolescence and young adulthood. Journal of Child Psychology and Psychiatry 46(8): 850-58.

Friedman, H. S., Tucker, J. S., Schwartz, J. E., et al. 1995. Childhood conscientiousness and longevity: Health behaviors and cause of death. Journal of Personality and Social Psychology 68(4): 696-703.

Hampson, S. E., Goldberg, L. R., Vogt, T. M., & Dubanoski, J. P. 2006. Forty years on: Teachers' assessments of children's personality traits predict self-reported health behaviors and outcomes at midlife. Health Psychology 25(1): 57-64.

———. 2007. Mechanisms by which childhood personality traits influence adult health status: Educational attainment and healthy behaviors. Health Psychology 26(1): 121-25.

Health Policy Brief. 2014. The relative contribution of multiple determinants to health outcomes. Health Affairs, August 21, 2014, described at www.healthaffairs.org/healthpolicybriefs/brief.php?brief_id=123, accessed 1/31/15.

Heckman, J. J. 2006. Skill formation and the economics of investing in disadvantaged children. Science 312(5782): 1900-2.

Howard, K. S., & Brooks-Gunn, J. 2009. The role of home-visiting programs in preventing child abuse and neglect. The Future of Children 19(2): 119-46.

Jackson, J. S., Knight, K. M., & Rafferty, J. A. 2009. Race and unhealthy behaviors: Chronic stress, the HPA axis, and physical and mental health disparities over the life course. American Journal of Public Health 100(5): 933-39.

Kulhánová, I., Hoffmann, R., Judge, K., et al. 2014. Assessing the potential impact of increased participation in higher education on mortality: Evidence from 21 European populations. Social Science and Medicine 117: 142-49.

Louie, G. H., & Ward, M. M. 2011. Socioeconomic and ethnic differences in disease burden and disparities in physical function in older adults. American Journal of Public Health 101(7): 1322-29.

Mani, A., Mullainathan, S., Shafir, E., & Zhao, J. 2013. Poverty impedes cognitive functioning. Science 341(6149): 976-80.

Michalopoulos, C., Lee, H., Duggan, A., et al. 2015. The Mother and Infant Home Visiting Program evaluation: Early findings on the Maternal, Infant, and Early Childhood Home Visiting Program. OPRE Report 2015-11. Washington, DC: Office of Planning, Research and Evaluation, Administration for Children and Families, US Department of Health and Human Services, available at www.acf.hhs.gov /programs/opre/resource/the-mother-and-infant -home-visiting-program-evaluation-early-findings -on-the-maternal-infant-and-early-childhood-home -visiting, accessed 3/5/15.

Moffitt, T. E., Arseneault, L., Belsky, D., et al. 2011. A gradient of childhood self-control predicts health, wealth, and public safety. Proceedings of the National Academy of Sciences USA 108(7): 2693-98.

National Academy of Sciences, Arthur M. Sackler Colloquium. 2011. Biological embedding of early social adversity: From fruit flies to kindergartners, described at www.nasonline.org/programs/sackler-colloquia /completed_colloquia/agenda-biological-embedding .html, accessed 8/22/14.

Reynolds, A. J., Richardson, B. A., Hayakawa, M., et al. 2014. Association of a full-day vs. part-day preschool intervention with school readiness, attendance, and parent involvement. JAMA 312(20): 2126-34.

Rigotti, N. A., Regan, S., Levy, D. E., et al. 2014. Sustained care intervention and postdischarge smoking cessation among hospitalized adults: A randomized clinical trial. JAMA 312(7): 719-28.

Rutter, M. 2012. Achievements and challenges in the biology of environmental effects. Proceedings of the National Academy of Sciences USA 109(Supp. 2): 17149-53.

Schwartz, J. E., Friedman, H. S., Tucker, J. S, et al. 1995. Sociodemographic and psychosocial factors in childhood as predictors of adult mortality. American Journal of Public Health 85(9): 1237-45.

Schweinhart, L. J. 2014. The value of high-quality full-day preschool. JAMA 312(20): 2101-2.

Schweinhart, L. J., Montie, J., Xiang, Z., et al. 2005. The High/Scope Perry Preschool Study through age 40: Summary, conclusions, and frequently asked questions. High/Scope Educational Research Foundation, available at www.highscope.org/file /specialsummary_rev2015_01.pdf, accessed 1/31/15.

Shariff-Marco, S., Klassen, A. C., & Bowie, J. V. 2010. Racial/ethnic differences in self-reported racism and its association with cancer-related health behaviors. American Journal of Public Health 100(2): 364-74.

Shaw, B. A., McGeever, K., Vasquez, E., Agahi, N., & Fors, S. 2013. Socioeconomic inequalities in health after age 50: Are health risk behaviors to blame? Social Science and Medicine 101: 52-60.

Wadden, T. A., Butryn, M. L., Hong, P. S., & Tsai, A. G. 2014. Behavioral treatment of obesity in patients encountered in primary care settings. JAMA 312(17): 1779-91.

Index

acculturation: definition of, 61; ethnic differences in, 61; patterns of, 61; racial discrimination and, 62

active life expectancy: association with disability level, 20; definition of, 19

Adler ladder of social position, 58

adolescence: cardiovascular disease in, 43; developmental changes in, 164-70; and early childhood intervention, 180-82

Adverse Childhood Experiences (ACE): Score, 156; Study, 156, 173

Adverse Childhood Experiences (ACEs): and childhood IQ score, 177; impact on child development, 173-74

Affordable Care Act, 116

Ainsworth, Mary, 111

allostatic load: association with behaviors, 44; and cognitive development, 178; cultural influences, 54; impact on adolescent behavior, 178; impact on child development, 152; role of hypothalamus, 131

American Academy of Pediatrics, 155; Council on Community Pediatrics, 184

American Psychological Association, 97, 136; research on motivation, 85

amygdala, 130; function of, 118; impact on executive function, 159-61; impact on hippocampus, 159; over-activity as a consequence of emotional stress, 159

anomie, definition of, 167

Apted, Michael, 89

arcuate fasiculus, 120-21, 139-40

assimilation, 61

association cortex, 125-26

Association of American Medical Colleges (AAMC), xiv

associative learning, 84-85, 118-21

attachment theory, 111-12

attention, 160-63

attitudes, 89-92, 165-70

attribution theory, 74-77; fundamental attribution error, 76-77

auditory cortex, role in the development of language, 123

auditory pathways in the brain, 118-21

auditory processing, 118-19

Austen Riggs mental health treatment center, 101

axon, brain, 118; development of, 122-24; myelination of, 123, 127-29

Bandura, Albert, 108

behavior: affected by presence of others, 77-79; association with preventable deaths, 35; attributing to persons or situations, 74-77; biological basis of, 115-32, 151-64, 173-79; brain and, 115-33; cognition and, 134-49; core components, 5; definition of, 2; environmental influences on, 63; motivation and, 82-96; normative and non-normative, 48-65; parental influence on, 48; personality and, 97-112; racial discrimination and, 63; social and cultural influences on, 48-65; social group membership, influence of, 68; social inequality and, 28-45, 151-70; steps in the process of, 115; and well-being, 11-26

Big Five Factor Structure, 104

Big Five Inventory, 105

Big Five personality traits, 8, 105-7; in different cultures, 106; ethnic differences, 61

biological basis of behavior, 115-32, 151-64, 173-79

biological factors: that affect cognition, 138-48, 156-64; in the regulation of motivation, 84-85

Birmingham Children's March (1963), 72

birth, premature, 13

Blumenbach, Johan, definition of races, 38

Bourdieu, Pierre, 68-69

Bowlby, John, 111

brain: association cortex, 125-26; and behavior, 115-33; functional units, 118; neural structure, 8; plasticity, 8, 132; stages in neuronal development, 124; structural arrangement, 117-21

Broca's area, 120-23, 139

bystander effect, 77-78

capital, alternative forms of, 68-69

cardiovascular disease in adolescence, racial and ethnic inequality in, 43

Carolina Abcedarian Project, 180-82

Carstensen, Laura, 92

Census, Canada, definition of races, 39

Census Bureau, U.S.: definition of ethnicity, 6, 37; definition of races, 6, 37-38

Center on Healthy, Resilient Children, 155

Centers for Disease Control and Prevention, U.S. (CDCP), 173, 179; components of well-being, 11; Health Disparities and Inequalities Report, 20, 30

Centers for Medicare and Medicaid Services, U.S., 116

central nervous system, 115-33

Childhood and Society (Erikson), 101

cigarettes. *See* smoking cigarettes

Civil Rights Act of 1964, 72